www.warriorarts.co.uk

MARA
SPS-67
SELF PROTECTION SYSTEM

TEN SQUARED
SECOND REVISION

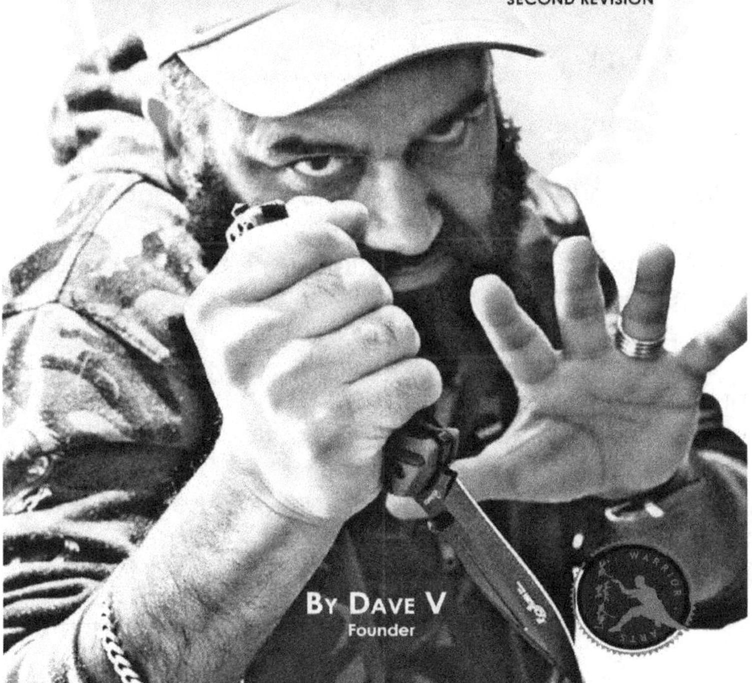

Forward

ISBN 978-1-9996712-0-4

The book is written in a relaxed, accessible and colloquial style. Those who have met Dave V, either personally or through his social media presence can hear him speak in his inimitable style, whilst those who do not, quickly get to know him.

The book brings a wealth of wisdom that is beneficial to the general public as well as martial arts practitioners.

This work is especially valuable for those who truly want to be effective in real-life encounters and might otherwise undertake 'martial arts' under the false belief that it will serve them on the street or other no-rules attack scenario.

Ten Squared is for everyone who wants to take their safety seriously, and gain some genuine and effective solutions to real street violence. It's equally for Martial arts enthusiasts who need to understand real violence, and effective techniques to counter it.

Ten Squared aims to address the following objectives:

To bring about a mind-set change about personal safety: becoming streetwise, perceptive, prepared and sensible.

To make you understand the true mentality of thugs and the idea that there is no 'fair fight'.

To give you a mindset, techniques and tools to be effective in real street fighting situations.

Introduction

Whilst we all know none of us are getting out of here alive, it is the definitive objective of this book to help you live a bit longer.

Think of martial arts and what do you think of? Bruce Lee? Kick boxing? Muay Thai? MMA? Grappling? High kicks? Karate suits? Silky robes? Ripped muscles?

My fundamental message in this book is that combat and real self-defence may not be best served by the well-known more commercial styles. Unless they are significantly augmented with specialist training, specialist knowledge and a specialist mindset. This can also sometimes be the case within the teaching of 'civilian derivatives' of well known military based self-defence styles.

This is all well-known to military combat trainers, who train elite specialist teams. Whilst they might pick and choose from the martial arts world to give them certain specialist skills, their overarching mindset and approach is very different from 'martial arts' - as we know them today.

Inevitably and purposely, movies and media desensitise us to the REAL impact of even a LITTLE bit of violence.
There is a certain sickening ugliness when even a little bit of actual violence goes down.

When people we know of get hurt, disabled or killed in a fight or attack from, for example, from a single blow to the head, or single stab wound, it shocks us to our core and our 'humanity' is deeply affected.

Martial arts classes can often compound the misconceptions about real violence. This occurs firstly in the combat SPORTS arena and secondly in the 'self-defence' arena.

Sports (generally) impose many constraints and many rules, they eliminate weapons and multiple opponent and operate in a direction, range and attitude that bares no resemblance to the reality of combat.

Self-defence and martial arts classes often utilise a fantasy version of the problem that is to be solved, for example, defence against a single technique, which could be an outstretched, static, punching arm or even worse an outstretched static knife-holding arm.

Real attacks are normally delivered from a stealthy position, often with a tirade of multi-angular blows or stabs in a whirlwind of unpredictable close range movement - delivered with intent and with an extreme sudden explosion of aggression.

This 'not knowing the question' and formulating answers to incorrect questions, often leaves practitioners of the martial arts in a worse position (in terms of real self-defence) than they were in prior to commencing their training.

At least they had their natural unmetered survival instincts intact prior to poor quality, misinformed training. Danger and risk occur when these primal instincts are replaced with new weakened reflexes.

Often beginners might possibly be better off investing in a heavy bag and simply pounding the hell out of it with bare fists, elbows, sticks and other weapons, all delivered with intent, rather than train in watered down derivatives of once potent arts.

The MARA Combat System has its' roots firmly in deadly ancient knowledge - but with a distinct modern flavour, it's faster to learn, makes the assumption that you might already have been hit or that you are outnumbered or are being attacked with a weapon, MARA is uncloaked, more accessible and contains methods that compensate for time. Time that we don't have. And chances we don't want to take.

After all, what good is a wonderful ancient advanced martial art - if you have to be a master with thirty years experience to use it? Similarly what use is one's highly effective combat art if it destroys the practitioner with injuries incurred whilst training and worse still whilst being demonstrated on by over-exuberant and often misinformed instructors. Misinformed in terms of the immediate and often delayed damage that ensue from strikes to pressure points on the head, neck and body. Yes they look good on YouTube ! But what of their students?

Real martial arts training should remind us how potentially fragile we all actually are.

Protecting yourself from the stark reality of violence and in turn exploiting these inherent weaknesses for your own genuine self-defence, is what full blooded combat is all about.

We also want to get a 'bigger bang for our buck' in combat, more from less effort and with more insurance policies for ourselves built in.

The ancient arts were brutal in the extreme, over the top by today's standards, in terms of lethality, deeply sinister, gut wrenchingly deadly, deceptive and secretive in layers that were hidden and unknown, even to adepts within the style. Often the inherent 'overkill' was to send a message to other would-be future attackers by building a dangerous reputation. Often 'reputation' alone is everything.

The meditative, breathing and energy building elements of the ancient arts were just as prolific as the martial teachings.

The objective of this book is to make you a better fighter, to eliminate as much fear and anxiety as possible, to make you calmer and more aware, more connected and more deadly; But only in honourable combat, where you genuinely consider your life or those around you might be endangered.

This book will help the beginner, advanced adept and instructor, to understand, practice and implement new ideas that will enhance ones combat ability tremendously.

Our genetics contain the genes of ancient warriors. The winners. The survivors. The hero's. The fighters. Feel that blood in your veins. Honour that blood. Stand tall. Stand strong. And don't be duped by the mass-media and the hype, as stated earlier, real combat is different to the movies and different to what's available in most martial arts classes.

If you have never done martial arts before or any kind of combat training, then this book should serve as an introduction in assisting you to finding a competent instructor and a worthy system. You'll learn some functional methods along the way. And yes this book will teach you about combat. It's not been written to be cryptic or hard to fathom.

If you are already training, then these pages should serve to stimulate thought and to enable you to augment and enhance your training and abilities in the sphere of real self-defence and real combat.

If you are an instructor, this book should hopefully enhance your teaching and personal understanding.

The techniques, ideas and methods in this book are dangerous and we accept no liability for death, injury or illnesses resultant. This book is for information purposes only, seek a competent and qualified instructor. The words lethal and deadly appear repeatedly in the book and have not been softened in favour of terms like 'neutralise' or 'stop' or 'defeat' etc. These stronger words were used on purpose, due to being more accurate and to act as a warning to all those that read this book, Martial Arts were originally deadly pursuits, any fighting, combat or defence is dangerous and can result in injury or death of one or more of the participants. If you can 'fight without fighting' then this is best, if you can avoid violence and prevent things from getting physical than this is also best.

A great saying is: Violence is rarely the solution, but when it is the solution it is the ONLY solution.

The Law.

The law varies country by country, state-by-state. Please appraise yourself of the moral, legal and ethical aspects of self-defence, weapons and improvised weapons where you live / operate.

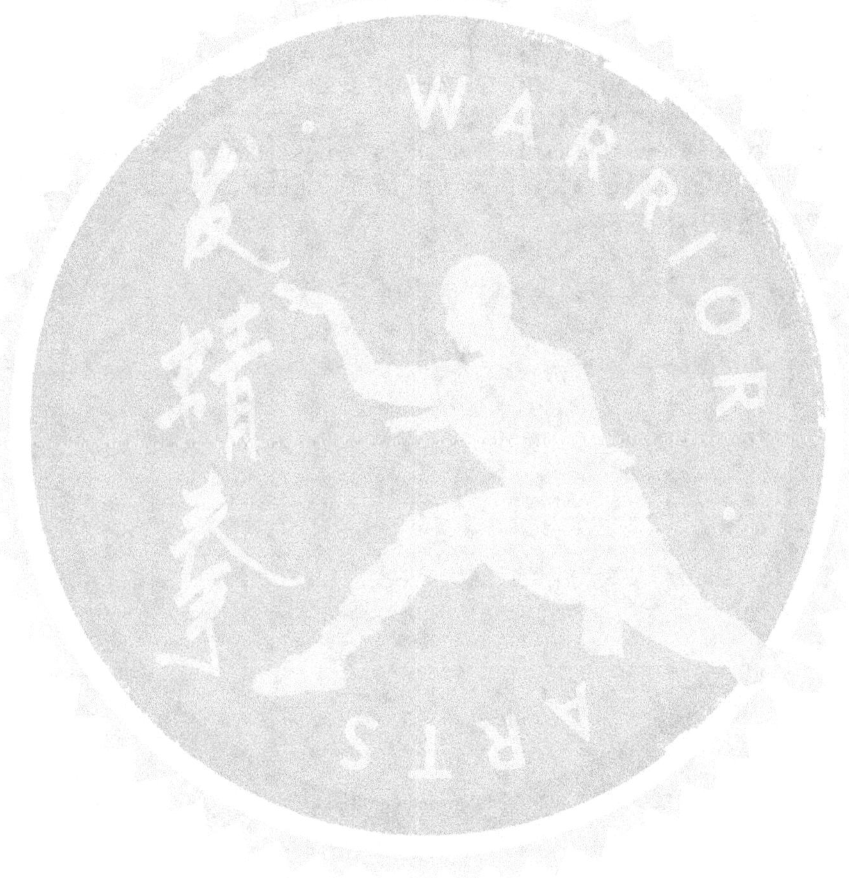

About Dave V.

Dave V started training in 1974, he holds multiple black belts and is the Founder of MARA Combat Systems. Dave has a Masters degree in computer science and information security and was a guest lecturer at the London Metropolitan Police Detective training school for 11 years. Qualified in advanced acupressure methods and with detailed knowledge of accu points and their application to fighting, Dave V has a voluminous knowledge on combat martial arts, deadly methods from ancient Dim Mak and extreme close range fighting. Dave V is well known on Instagram, with many world wide followers to his daily self-defence tips, colourful language, helpful life advice and antidotes.

Check out warriorarts.co.uk for more info on Dave, his lineage and the arts he studied.

MARA encompasses a branch of extreme martial arts and practices, that embody ultra-close range combat, advanced and dangerous pressure point and vital point strikes, explosive energy power development and weapons (conventional and improvised) application. MARA is a reflexive art that seeks to capitalise on natural body responses, which are tweaked and re-embedded to create a more prolific combat response.

MARA is based on ancient Chinese arts, which have been seamlessly blended with military methods and modern fight science. The objective being to up your chances in real high pressure situations.

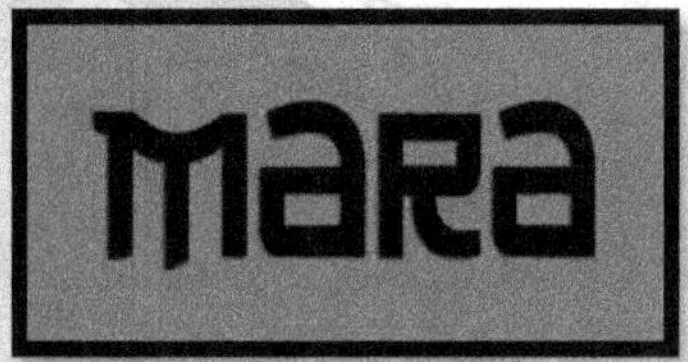

The ancient animal styles also lend heavily into MARA - mainly from the Monkey, Tiger and Snake. These give the entry methods, the clawing and the elusive speed. Finally, the ancient drunken boxing methods have been embedded to give the unpredictable, deceptive and shocking pre-emption that epitomises the style.

The internal or meditational element of the training is equal to the martial aspect in terms of emphasis, importance and time spent.

Many modern combat arts now utilise various deceptive guard positions, head guard entries and rapid clawing. But the ancient roots of these are well known and recognised in MARA. Dave V spend over twenty years learning these ancient arts and 15 years teaching them.

Contents

One - The Mind.

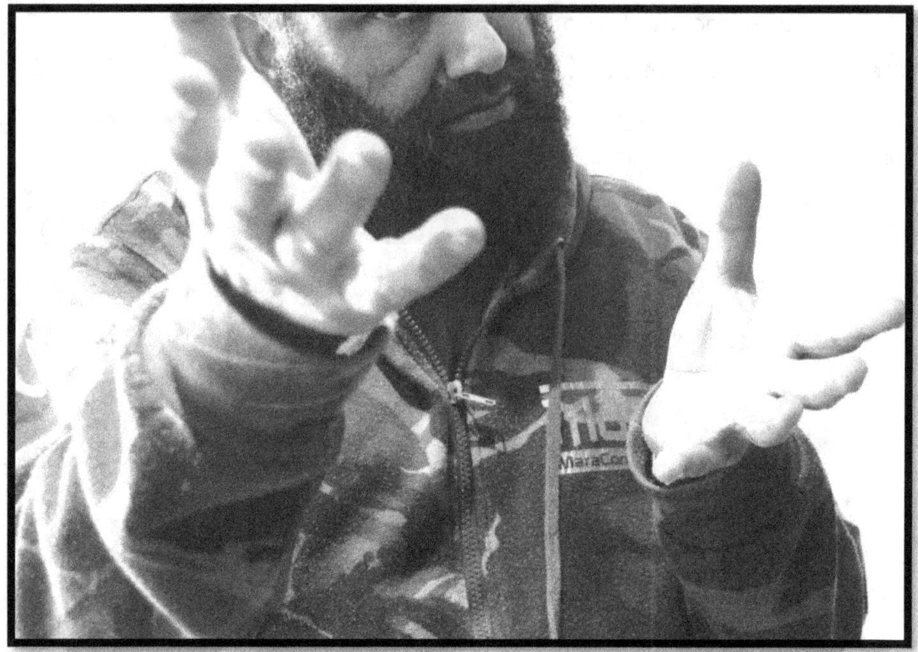

I.   Their motives, the attack and your survival

People's motives for attacking civilians (civilians = debt loaded, law abiding, tax paying consumers, diligent workers, good and obedient civilians, who have been willing parties to the normalisation process and who are happily compliant, hopeful, placid and unarmed), range from sexual attack, drink or drugs related violence and anger, taking personal possessions, whether at home or on the street or road rage et cetera.

If your lifestyle necessitates that you must rub shoulders with the criminal class, then revenge can also often play a part in violence, as can 'disrespect' and gang related violence. Or simply being in the wrong place at the wrong time.

Understand your 'value', what you have and what people might want. Understand your behaviour and the need for avoidance, prevention, de-escalation and sensitivity in certain situations.

What are the main risk points in our lives? Is it relationships? going out? Bars? Parking? Home security? The areas we live? Walking our dogs? Running late at night or in lonely places? ....or is it our own lack of awareness or our sometimes 'unfortunate manner' that tends to aggravate people?

Attacks can occur outside, inside, by strangers or people you know. There is normally some sort of lead up, attacker preparation, in particular a physical and psychological 'gearing up'. Observe and become familiar with how people 'change'. How their eyes, posture and voice often change and how they become jerky and then still just prior to attack.

You can and must survive.

Stopping things before they start or preventing an escalation, are your best strategies. These few seconds could be the most critical of your life. So be prepared for the worst and hope for the best.

II.   Understanding violence

Some people do it for power and control. Others for money. Others to show off. And some because they are drunk or high.

Some people are opportunists and other plan every move. In any event, people who are violent often start small and increase their thrill. In domestic situations have zero tolerance as it will almost ALWAYS get worse as sociological studies have shown.

Some people operate normally and only get violent when drink or drugs are added to the mix.

Some people are pathological, sick and twisted, some people have grown up with violence and violent behaviour has simply become the norm.

Living in a so-called civilised society means that we can't simply eliminate or erase society members who have caused us harm. Instead, it seems, they need to be 'understood' 'empathised' with and treated specially or rehabilitated to help them. If they are sometimes caught (by the highly motivated but under-funded and under-resourced law enforcement industry), then the often low-level penalties for injuring innocent people or even killing, can seem very lenient to the victims and families.

You are not a victim or a willing participant. You deserve to be safe and sound and you have a legal right to defend yourself (within the law), your loved ones and your property.

The police are good at their jobs, especially in picking up (or moping up) the pieces, cordoning off the area and drawing chalk lines. It's very unlikely they will be there when you get attacked.

Leave nothing to chance, take charge of your own safety and that of your loved ones.

III.   Victim v Predator

The law of the jungle denotes who is predator and who is the prey. Which are you? We need to strive to be assertive and confident but when needed we have to be able to 'switch' and become even more predatory than those who seek to harm us.

This gives the attacker a shock as they realise INSTINCTIVELY that they have misjudged you. Your size doesn't matter. It's how 'controlled crazy' you can become that matters. It's what your eyes say, what your body says, what your face says.

IV.   The human, The Brain, The Animal

So, it turns out we have different types of brains in our head. A calm poetic, creative and spiritual human brain. And various brain levels beneath this. Deep, deep below this, we have an animalistic brain, this controls our automatic functions, like breathing and heartbeat. This stuff lives in the medulla oblongata. The brain stem. It is this anatomical friend that can fight AUTOMATICALLY and with potentially DEADLY affect when necessary and appropriate. If we know how to let 'him' take over and do his job.

The logical, compassionate and poetic part of the brain does not generally win fights (to defend us when attacked) .

V.   Mental training

Who do you know that is vulnerable, old, disabled, young, weak? Choose one person. Hopefully you love them. Imagine them being attacked by a crazed individual or a gang. Only you stand between them and death. What would you do to defend them? What mind-set would you need? Practice this feeling.

Feel this feeling. Awaken this feeling. Feel the passion and blood pounding through you. We need to harness and harvest this energy.

VI. Physical training

Exhaust yourself, run, do bag work, do serious circuits, then do three one-minute rounds of all-out milling on the pads or bag, that means anything goes, work through the torture of fatigue and harness the mental thoughts and visualisation created in the previous section.

VII. Awakening and training the Animal

Develop a word, an expression, a posture and a hand position, that embodies and expresses the 'Animal mode' within you. This is the bridge between 'normal you' and 'animal you'. My students open their eyes, curve their back and open their 'claws'. They might also growl and snarl. Train the animal to obey and also to be free to do his job.

VIII. Peace and tranquility v anxiety

You will not be able to fight in animal-mode if you suffer from anxiety.

Anxiety is the polite, civilised and modern word for FEAR.

Learn about breathing and Chinese energy work, also known as Qi Gong, these methods teach you to breathe properly.

If you have correct posture and breathing, it will not only allow you into animal-mode easier but will also let the energy flow for self-healing.

The net result can be a marked decrease in anxiety.

Also clean up your diet, go Paleo and avoid all intoxicants, as this also fuels anxiety.

Finally, live a life congruent with who you are, avoid jobs / careers that 'stress you out', don't be a square peg in a round hole, get on a course and retrain or open your own business. Be brave. Getting stressed and bullied at work is never worth it. Understand, that to them, you're totally and utterly expendable. If you have a stress induced stroke or cardiac arrest – your boss is NOT going to look after your family.

IX.   Understanding stress

Like anxiety, stress is often resultant from fear. Stress can be healthy - if we use it properly as a trigger or motivator, but in our modern age it's often toxic. The massive amounts of adrenaline dumping into the system for fight or flight never gets used because you're sitting down in the office or bickering with a partner and the result is we get stressed.

Inevitably this leads to learned behaviours and responses - depression is normally the result.

Here's the normal pattern. Anxiety - Stress - Depression.

Often people self-medicate with legal highs, i.e. highly taxed alcohol and/or illegal drugs, or hanker for meaningless entertainment from the media. Ironically, certain natural herbs were in every hypothecary i.e. Middle Ages pharmacy, because they helped with anxiety, stress, melancholia and mania. These natural herbs and many other traditional herbs are now generally illegal and instead people who have a genuine need, often have to substitute with illegally grown and unnaturally altered, imbalanced strains of various 'herbs', which don't have any medicinal property, only a garish and undesirable hallucinating affect... which is in itself often addictive and self-destructive.

X.   Relaxed killer mindset, the calm in the centre of the storm

Real Martial Arts / Combat training enables you to stay calm and use the 'no-minded' state during the heat of combat. Your animal brain takes over and your human mind is protected. At the end of the altercation you will not know exactly what you did because your animal brain reflexively did what was necessary, through its' proper learned responses, i.e. those contained within this book.

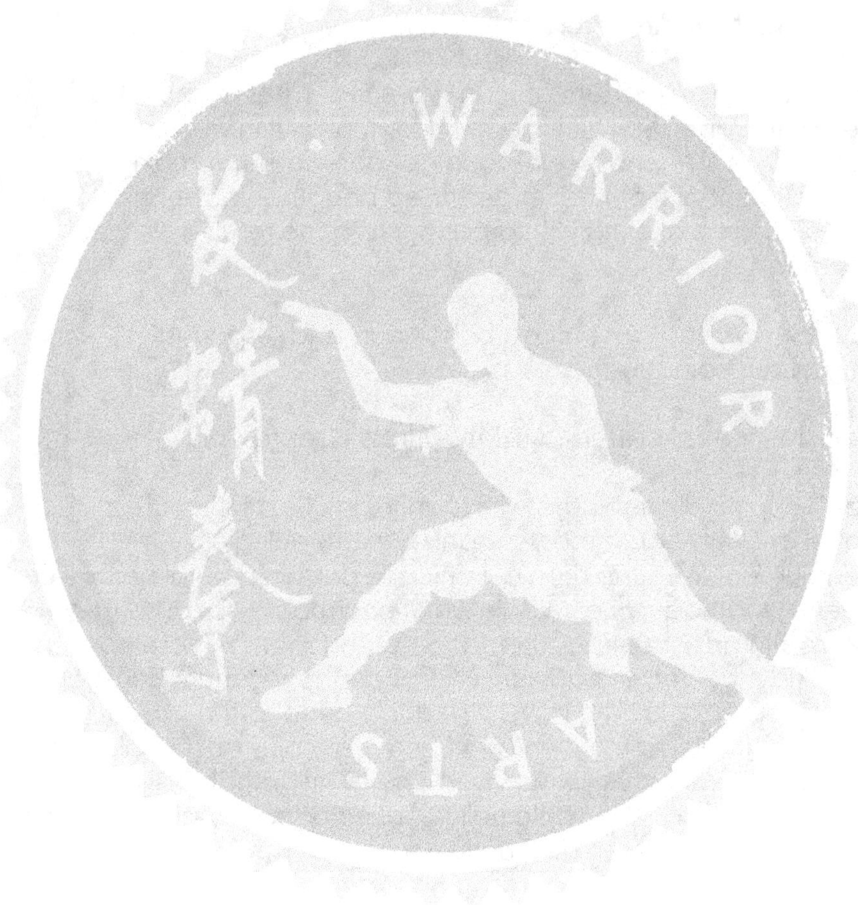

Two - Awareness, tunnel vision, peripheral vision

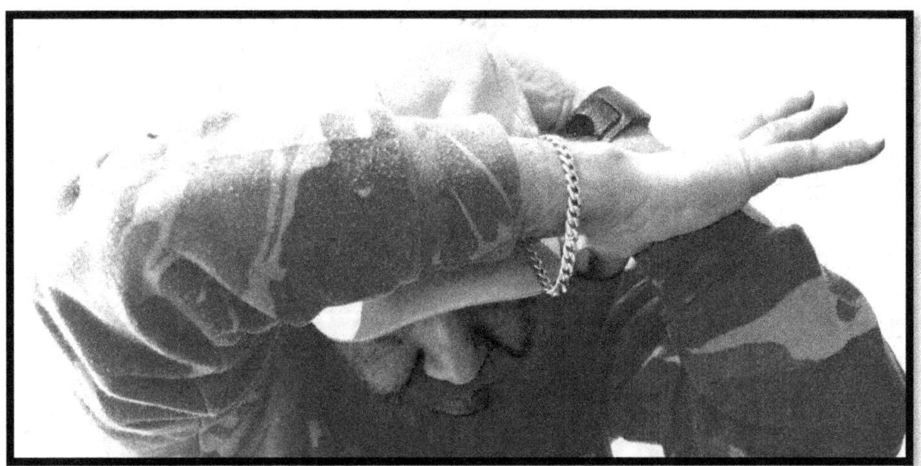

I. How to get killed, robbed, attacked, molested.

Here are 15 ways to increase the chances of being attacked:

Don't read the signs that situations are becoming dangerous.

Walk around with your head down on your phone, whilst staring at the pavement.

Make sure you walk, run, jog, through lonely places that are dark or dimly lit. With your Head phones in.

Park your car in the most dangerous place, e.g. rough areas or dark carparks.

Do not plan ahead for safety when you go to new places.

Go places where people like to drink a lot and stay there well into the early hours until people have lost all control of their minds.

If you are a woman - go on Internet dates with people you are not sure about and if they do not look like theIR picture and start to behave oddly - stay with them anyway and accept a lift home.

Leave your children with neighbours or friends you don't know well.

Have no awareness of your own behaviour and be rude to people who might have a short fuse and who might be inclined to violence.

Wander cluelessly into the wrong area or gang-controlled areas.

Have no awareness in high risk areas such as airports, travel terminuses, busy shopping areas, packed bars and nightclubs.

Leave your drink unattended and take random unlicensed cabs home.

Start to feel happy and comfortable when you turn into your road and have no awareness of who is behind you when you put the keys in the door.

Let anyone with an ID badge or uniform into your home.

When people are gearing up for violence, act passively and hope for pity.

II.   How not to get killed, robbed, attacked, molested

Take note of the paragraph above! And do the opposite.

In all seriousness, have your wits about you, plan for the worst and hope for the best. Do at least some reconnaissance in terms of new areas you're visiting, be they locally or internationally. Let common sense prevail and take your personal security seriously. In particular, train the elderly people and other vulnerable people in your family on how to avoid the risks outlined above.

III.   How to be aware

Retrain your behaviour and your eyes to look around and be prepared to take alternative routes or to simply avoid places and people which may be hostile.

Develop strategies to extricate yourself from situations and places. Do not worry about upsetting people or hurting their feelings, your safety is more important. If they are genuine then they will not be upset or hurt. Do not simply stumble into situations, people, groups of people - if you feel they may be the slightest chance of danger, then take evasive action.

IV.   Mental training for effective peripheral vision

Animals instinctively use their peripheral vision and see a much wider detailed picture than we do. We tend to become very tunnel visioned most of the time. Animals are only tunnel visioned when they are about to strike, pounce, attack or kill.

When you are out and about, walking or on the bus or train, look straight ahead and use your **mind** to look left, right, up and down. Absorb the widest picture you can and train that part of your mind which we rarely use. Make this your default position. Once you have mastered this level, learn to focus in on certain people or objects whilst simultaneously training your peripheral vision, this will train your full vision even more deeply. This will be most beneficial to you in avoiding situations and people well before they get near to you. Augment this practice with regular scanning of the most distant area in front, the immediate foreground, the sides and also behind you

V.   Understanding and awareness regarding the prelude to violence

There is normally a prelude. This means there is normally a warning. This could be from someone following you and speeding up or mirroring your direction of travel, or someone's body language or eyes changing. Typically, there is a calm before the storm. Typically, people try to cloak their intention and the fact they are getting within range of attacking you, by using verbal distraction and / or moving their limbs in certain ways which seem normal...until they pounce, grab, strike, kick or attack in a variety of ways.

VI.   Physical training solo

Watch videos on YouTube of real attacks and familiarise yourself of the preludes alluded to here. Learn some more too. Familiarity with violence and it's preludes will assist you greatly in spotting it. When you interact with people understand the different ranges where they could or could not attack you. Always seek to be out of range with strangers. Learn to continually and naturally alter your distance and always be wary of people who would not allow you to affect and maintain your comfortable distance.

VII. Physical training partner

Work with a partner and get them to talk and threaten whilst out of range and then get them to move in randomly. Get used to the way they move in. Work different angles and even from behind. Progressively increase the partner training so that you move out of range initially, but then change the training so you move into them as they seek to enter your space, this is combat ! Investigate moving in at different angles.If they wish to be close, you get closer and deadlier ! The final stage of training is to actually unleash a flurry of your own attacks when they are planning to enter your space, by moving in and attacking ! preferably with them wearing a head guard and body armour.

VIII. Physical training pads

As above but unleashing your attacks onto various training equipment like pads and shields, this will enable you to go full power without the worry of hurting your training partner.

IX.   On the street

Be aware that people may bump into you, in order to elicit a hostile response, whereby they can justify attacking you. Their friends maybe be videoing the incident, which has been orchestrated in order to knock you out for entertainment. Always cross the road when you see a gang, dodgy group or street drinkers. Cross the road well before or take a different route. In this day and age it is pretty straight forward to turn around and get to safety whereupon one can call an Uber cab, which is normally there within minutes.

X.   In other high-risk areas, airports, whilst travelling, in bars, approaching home, entering vehicles etc.

Be aware that a lot of abductions, robberies and violence tend to occur in the above areas. In particular, people are very vulnerable when they approach home or their vehicle because they feel they are about to enter a safe area. Attackers know that peoples guard is often down when they put the key into the door of their house or vehicle. One does not need to explain what could happen next...

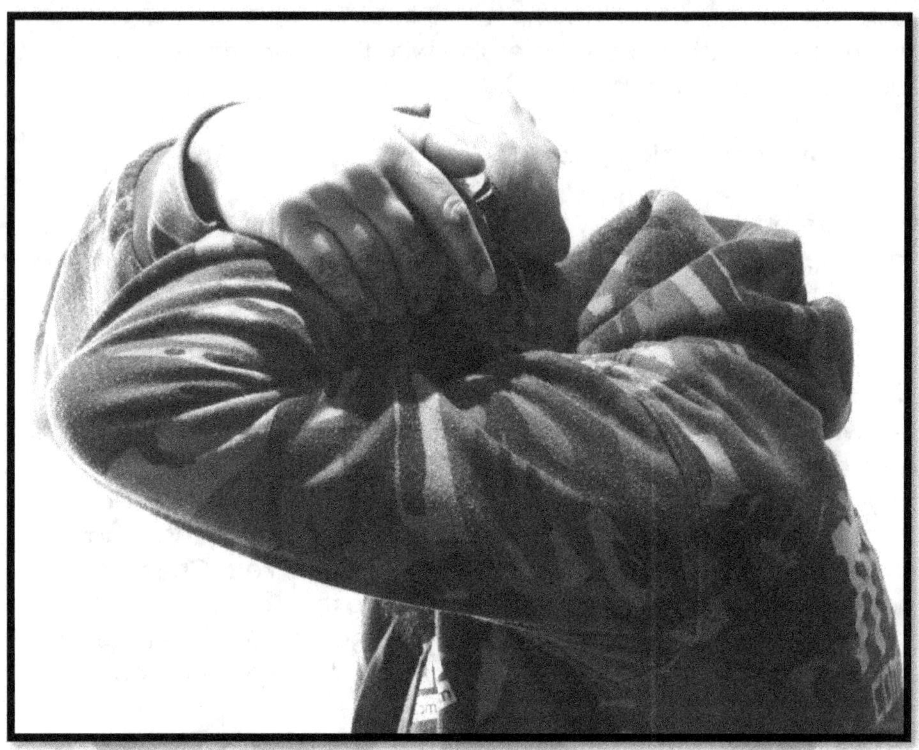

I.   **Dating.**

London Metropolitan police have posted a bulletin in bars and various other establishments warning people about the dangers of dating in terms of feeling uncomfortable, date rape drugs and also people not being who they say they are. They have a campaign called 'Ask for Angela', whereby worried patrons can go to the bar and ask for help and a taxi to safety. Vet any prospective people you are due to meet, checking them out on social media, their internet presence and the details of their profile generally. Ensure that their profile has not been cut-and-pasted from elsewhere and that any meetings are in a public place, where your friends and family know where you are. Prevention is better than cure. Never leave the establishment with someone you feel uncomfortable with and never meet someone in a lonely, secluded place without help nearby. If attacked use stealth and timing to affect a telling pre-emptive strike thus enabling your escape. If the attacker is much bigger than you or the threat is deadly / serious, arm yourself with an improvised weapon or blunt object of some type and strike with full commitment to affect your escape.

II.   Multiple attackers

The general rule in multiple attackers situations, which develop quickly, is to attack pre-emptively (if you cannot escape) at the most aggressive of the attackers. Use stopping power to affect a strategy of 'shock and awe' in order to deter the other attackers and to make them feel you are 'crazy' and don't care about getting hurt in your zeal to fight them. Avoid being in the middle of the pack.

Use the proper covert entry methods, which protect your most vulnerable areas and attack their most vulnerable areas.

Timing is everything as is using your most dangerous body weapons, to focus the biggest power to the smaller surface area or hardest bony surface know how to use your body as a weapon.

Again, the use of improvised weapons (or <u>self defence tools</u> where the law allows) for example umbrellas, sticks, bricks, stones, dirt, keys, phones and anything else at hand, will be in an invaluable aid to your escape, success and survival.

Use a stance that is balanced so if you are attacked from the rear you won't easily fall over or you may also use this good stance to throw people over your shoulder. If you are taken to the ground then bite, scratch, rip, gauge and use any illicit, banned and dirty method to get up as quickly as possible. Learn to kick with great ferocity from the ground into the assailants knee, groin et cetera.

III.   Burglary

Take sensible preventative steps, get an alarm, if you are female living on your own have a pair of large men's work boots in your porch way or first thing as you enter. Get a dog or get an alarm that makes the sound of a dog barking or at the least have a warning sign about a dog.

Leave lights on when you are out, have lights on a timer, leave the radio or television on so there is sound. Use technology to best effect with covert cameras with remote IP login. This should all be linked to an alarm system. An alarm box outside with a light flashing serves as a good deterrence. Neighbourhood watch schemes and good relationships with neighbours are also essential in preventing burglary. Planting thorny bushes to the rear to prevent climbing in and extending the height of fences also acts as suitable barriers and defence. Trimming back shrubbery, plants and trees from the front area will remove hiding places and ambush zones. Fitting powerful light sensors to the front side and rear which go off when triggered will also make inhospitable territory for the burglar. Putting down sharp shingle/gravel to any entrance points also serve to deter burglars due to the crunching noise resultant. Leave the keys to any vehicles, especially attractive vehicles where they can be easily found near the main access point. This will avoid the dangerous necessity of the burglar coming upstairs in the hunt for keys. Train yourself in the use of weapons (check the law where you are) or improvised weapons, have a variety of these handy. In certain countries this may be a firearm in other countries this may be a taser in other countries this may be a simple combat stick, it might also be an umbrella, a knife or anything that you have at hand. Ensure that you and your love ones know the whereabouts of all covert and improvised weaponry in the household. They should be strategically and covertly placed in case of intruders.

Ensure all bedrooms have internal locking systems in case of break in into the main areas. This will serve to protect children and the vulnerable. Some intruder systems will allow you to place the downstairs on a separate loop, so that intruders can be detected and alarms raised early.

Train yourself in the use of weaponry and use the elements of surprise to launch a pre-emptive attack.

Train all family members in how to raise the alarm, how to raise calls to emergency services and what to say. Ensure all family members understand that even making a silent call to the emergency services will normally result in a Police Officer being called out more often than not.

In countries where the law is strict and burglars have "rights", consider training to maim but not kill - e.g. by striking to the legs with power kicks or blows with sticks, truncheons or other improvised implements. However, for many a good general rule is that it is better to be judged by a jury rather than be carried by coffin bearers.

IV. Robbery

Developing proper awareness and implementing basic anti-surveillance strategies are essential. At a basic level, not having one's head down and texting is always a good idea !

Anti-surveillance is an advanced art but basically involves spotting those planning malevolent acts against you, who might be watching you or your property with intent, setting you up, or actually following you....and closing in.

Keeping away from dimly lit, lonely areas is a good plan, equally important is not allowing familiarity to lull you into a sense of false security. Criminals often wander instinctively into areas where there are rich picking, where victims are perceived as weak office workers with laptops, devices and expensive phones.

Train in the use of improvised weapons, like keys, pens, phones, umbrellas and other handy implements. If you live in a country where covert or overt weapons are allowed - then train in the effective drawing and automatic reflexive use of these.

For unexpected rear attacks understand that one needs to adopt a totally different approach to normal combat...this normally involves advanced stand up grappling, the use of unorthodox rear striking methodology and a definitive need for improvised weaponary to level the playing field or stack the odds more in your favour.

V.   Molestation / Sexual Attacks

Most of these attacks are likely to be carried out by people you know or have just met. In rare circumstances these might be out and out attacks on the street and in the home, affected by stealth entry.

For the former be wary and listen to your gut and adopt sensible rules of conduct for women and children in your family. Basically, leave them unsupervised with other males at your peril. For rape sitations, prepare to fight and flee, inflict fight stopping damage to the eyes, throat, groin and other vital points, using sharp improvised objects such as lip pens, hairbrushes, hair pins, failing that...bite, gauge, tear, use elbows, hammer fists and knees, do the worst damage you can in a single surprise explosion, precede this with mock momentary fear / compliance trickery, if the situation demands that and you have no choice. Then affect telling blows, strikes or use improvised weapons methods and flee to safety and report matters to the police either whilst fleeing or when at safety.

VI. Kids

Bully proof your children with a good upbringing, disciplined and
respectful with plenty of boundaries, reward and punishment.
Martial arts training should start early, choose something practical,
like kick boxing, wrestling, maybe JKD or MARA for kids. Make sure
they have proper anti-abduction training.

Steer clear of martial arts grading factories that cost the earth but
where it's just a commercial belt that is awarded. One way to break
their martial interest is to get them a commercial black belt that
they know has zero value on the street. Invest in their training
properly. Get advice from a combat expert if needed. If their
martial art doesn't cover multiple attackers, use of elbows and
knees or head butts and doesn't teach them about abduction
prevention and methodology.....then it isn't a martial art that's fit for
today's purpose. Or any purpose for meaningful combat.

Do not break their spirit by constant brow beating, undermining and
well meaning hand holding and mollycoddling. If you have a boy
then train him to be a man. Education is important but not as
important as being a strong, assertive man. Make your boy
Alpha....or his life will be very hard indeed. Don't emasculate.
Empower and make him a warrior for all life's trials and tribulations.

Every child needs to know how to defend themselves, how to stay
out of danger and harm, how to deal with stranger danger, how to
disable a larger opponent, flee the scene and call for help.

VII. Travelling

Airports, travel terminus, bus stations, rail stations. These places
represent danger as they often attract beggars, druggies, vagrants
and various desperadoes. These places are often warm, sheltered
and have rich pickings of hundreds / thousands of transient people,
often distracted and / or excited about their destinations and travel.
These people are often laden with goodies, devices, gifts, ID

documents, cash and cards. These days we can add to the mix that pretty young people often travel alone or with other equally pretty and often clueless compadres. The potential pickings are rich in all regards. From overt hold ups, to stealth pick pocketing, to bags going missing and people disappearing from taking taxis and other lifts from other 'travellers' they have met.

The solutions include awareness, effective counter surveillance methods, operated at an instinctive and automatic level and a healthy ability to say no and to fend off approaches, conversations and attempts to talk, from ANY stranger. Setting phones on a family mapping group is also a good idea, so that geo location is possible if someone goes missing.

Encourage female travel companions to visit the toilet with someone else when travelling in strange locations. Either send another female or stand outside the toilet and wait. Also get them to check the safety of the toilet area and immediately report back to you before using the facilities. Also train females to quickly scan for covert cameras and to cover any gaps that could hide such devices. The proliferation of covert camera and recording devices is massive, as is the probable increase in the number of perverts, peados and sickos of various types - check the internet and see for yourself what's available in terms of mini hidden cameras !

VIII. Opening the door

One of the biggest dangers for the elderly, young and vulnerable is opening the front door of their safe enclosure to those from the outside world.

We need to prevent, deter, discern and deal with those whom may have malevolent intent, mental disturbances which make them dangerous and those who are rendered dangerous, desperate and unpredictable due to drugs and drink.

We also need to train our loved ones to prevent opening the door

to the mentally ill sexual predators or people who are simply evil minded. This is a challenge when so many delivery men now operate for our growing internet shopping culture.

Invest in overt electronic cameras as deterrence. This means your dependents no longer have to come to the door, invest in a speaker and IP camera / bell system. Vet everyone. If your premises is sufficiently large, then invest in a gated system, whereby all would be callers wait at the perimeter.

Dogs are a great deterrence. Full stop. Get the right one and train it to bark and protect. Do not stifle it's natural guarding and pack instinct.

ID cards mean nothing. Only allow entry to pre arranged callers. Never open the gates or doors to those alleging an emergency pertaining to phone lines, water leaks, gas leaks, utilities etc.

Even those from the emergency services are to be treated with healthy suspicion and proper checks should be made to confirm their legitimacy.

In our society the elderly often live on their own, even after their spouse has passed away. This often leaves them very vulnerable to callers, alleged emergencies and 'urgent' remedial building work where costs spirals out of control. This is a sad reality. Protect your older relatives. Build an independent granny flat and keep them on your premises if at all possible.

Keep a keen eye on the finances of your teenage dependents and elderly parents. Spot exploitation early and call the police for help and guidance. Confront criminals if you are able and let them know you are wise to their scams.

Use a chain to open the door. Fit a spy hole.

Keep an improvised weapon nearby.

IX. Alcohol

Booze is an intrinsic element of life in the West. It's an intrinsic part of many aspects of life, relationships and society and is used in order to relax, celebrate, commiserate, and socialise. Many people are occasional or social drinkers and no significant harm to self or others is done.

There is however a school of thought that alcohol should be a class A drug. For many who can't control it, it's addictive in the extreme, can destroy health, wealth, relationships and family and can turn a normal person into a very unpleasant version of themselves.

Initially, it's a euphoric and a stimulant and a remover of inhibitions. It can feel good. If more and more is consumed, then the inevitable downward cycle sets in. The slowing down of mental faculties, the confusion of mind and thought and then drunkenness and sickness. People can get into fights over nothing, insult people, sleep with people they didn't intend to sleep with and commit violence and sexual assaults which would not have been otherwise committed, due to the inhibitory centre of the brain not operating effectively and putting the brakes on. In certain age groups, cultures or socio economic groups, binge drinking is the norm and is a right of passage, the evidence of a 'good night out' or a sign of 'manliness'.

If you want to be safer, stay away from places where people congregate to drink. If you have to be in these places then be alert to people who are drunk, over exuberant, shouting or who start staring at you.

High Level skilled martial artists often don't drink, we have a bigger responsibility to stay in control. And we may get into worse trouble with the law if we overreact. It's also soul destroying (and embarrassing) when a person who has dedicated their life to martial arts and combat, can't defend themselves or their loved ones because they are drunk!

X.   Car parks

Extra vigilance is required.

Carrying heavy shopping, taking lifts and walking into blind alleys and wandering around dimly lit carparks, can all be a clear invitation to criminals and attackers. Park on the street and pay a bit extra.

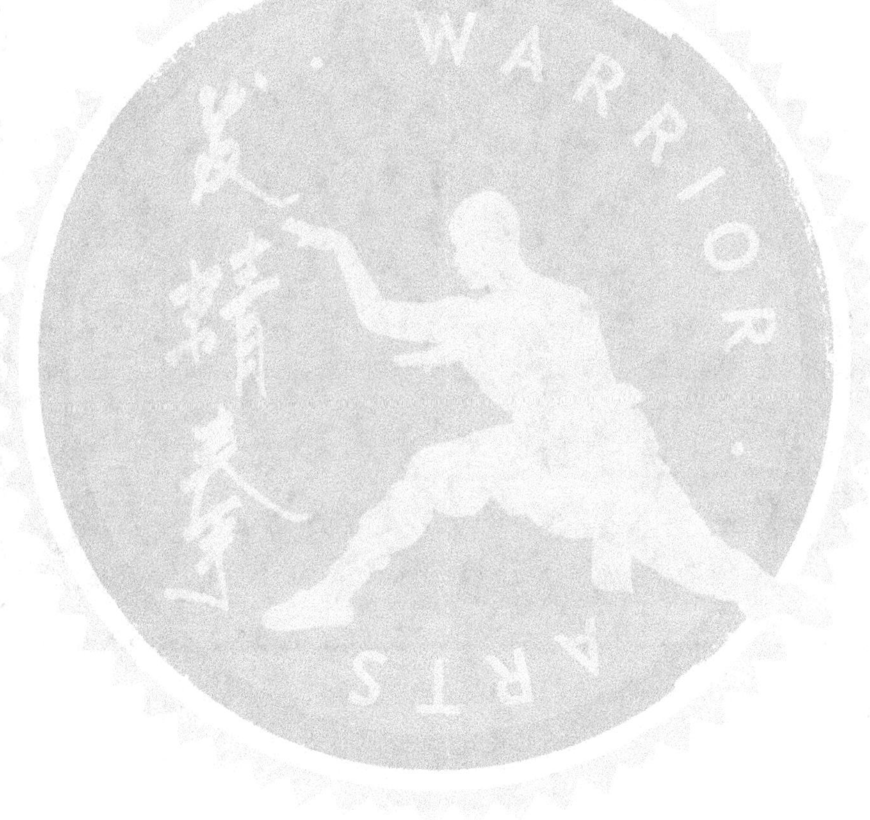

Four - Pre Emption

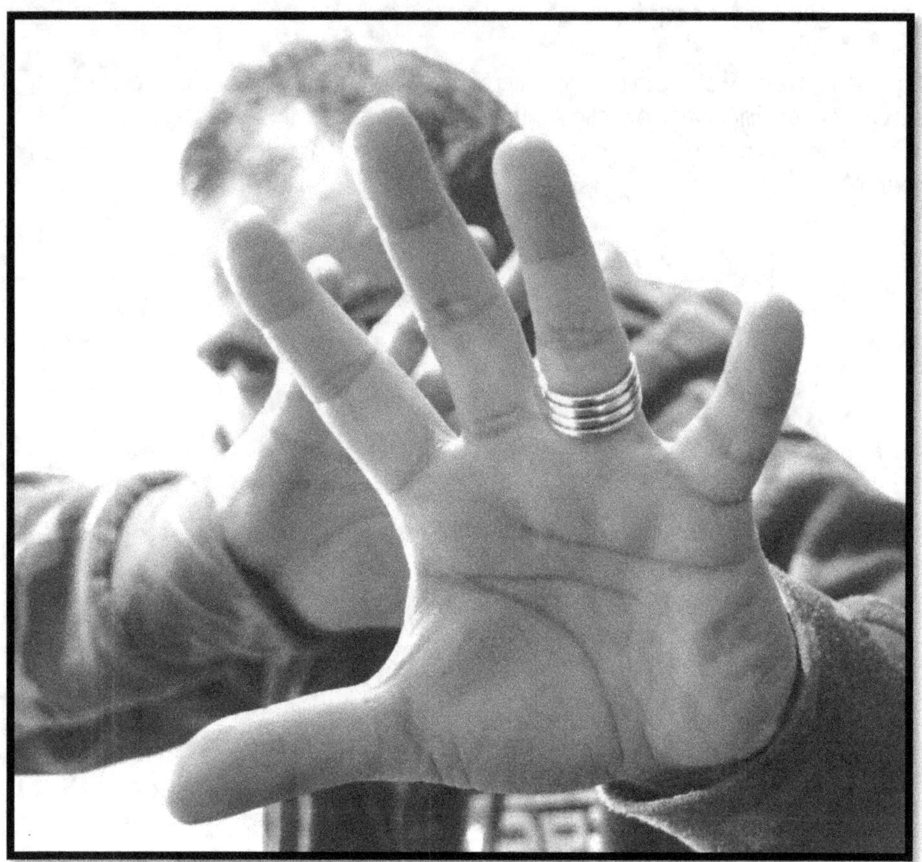

I.   Why

Blocks don't work.

Being defensive doesn't tend to work either.

If you wait for your attacker or attackers to take the initiative and attack you first, your misplaced moral high ground and flawed training concepts could get you beaten up or dead.

In full-blooded combat a pre-emptive approach is the one which is generally favoured.

Hit first, hit hard, hit to finish, inflict a surprise attack where the prey (you) becomes the predator - in a heartbeat.

II.   When to attack

Here are some classic times to launch your pre emptive attack:

Whilst 'talking it down'
Whilst seeming to comply
Whilst moving in a broken rhythm
When they least expect it
Before they move
Before they strike
When they think you are weak
In that moment when the pack are gaining their collective drive to move as a wave against you.

III.   How

With full commitment
Without hesitation
With proper training and weaponry behind you
Proper weaponry which can be empty handed, improvised or conventional
Focusing the most power into an explosive, unexpected strike that implants the most power into the smallest, hardest, sharpest or bluntest weapon, dependent upon the technique you are using and / or the target you are homing in on.
With a hammer fist, sharp elbow, shoulder, eye strike, head butt, sharp body blow, your keys, umbrella or any other implement.

IV. Solo training

Launch slowly and smoothly for a multitude of different angles, with a number of favourite unarmed, armed and improvised weapons. This gets you to bond with your weapons and find the groove.

Then speed up the above.

Then speed it up more.

Then make it explosive,

Then add intent.

V. Partner training

All the above but done with partner/s, also add body shields and helmets, so that an element of realism enters the mind of both the attacker and the victim, who is about to become the predator. There should always be a ramification for you in getting it wrong !

Partner training can then steadily progress from one partner to two to many. The training should start slow and build confidence and technique, until sufficient competence has been gained to enter the pressure test arena, where things get as real as they can get in training.

VI. Pads and shields

Then add shields, pads, tyres (to strike with sticks) and whatever else you can get to practice striking with unrestrained power and commitment.

Place the pads and shields at different angles to replicate all the single and multiple attacker scenarios you can think of. Start off stationary, then get the pads to move in from being just out of range. Start with medium power and work up to full power in these

pre arranged set sequences. Once these have been trained and proficiency gained, move onto unorchestrated scenarios by placing the shields and pads randomly and at will of the pad holders. Safety is important, don't hit the pad holders !
Also get your partners to bundle you to the ground and learn to strike and kick the shields and pads from the ground ! Then get up and carry on striking !

Motivate the 'man in middle' to strike with power, commitment and tenacity and beast them to gain confidence and resilience and this rather extreme training mode.

VII. Distancing

Correct distancing i.e. closing the distance, especially when achieved through deceptive and covert means, will double the impact and efficacy of any pre emptive blow or strike. Trick your enemy with the surprise delivery of an explosive fingertip eye strike, where the victim attacker may feel (subconsciously) that they are out of range and are therefore safe.

Attack by draw, where you invite an attack by creating an opening, this is an advanced methid and is a risky business and not recommended for multiple attacker life or death combat.

Basically, teach yourself to talk, play the victim, play the predator, distract, strike whilst talking, strike whilst moving in, strike whilst moving out, strike using finger tips to create elusive reach and finally internalise snake-like flowing explosive movements that are hard to predict. Be non telegraphic and generally elusive and shocking.

VIII. Strikes, ranges, targets and weapons

Some favourite strikes to work for preemption are:

Head guard elbows.
Head butts.
Hammer fist strikes
Thumb strikes to eyes
Finger tip strikes to eyes or neck
Palms
Shoulder strikes
Downwards elbow tip strikes over the guard
Various armed and improvised weapons.

Clearly, the distance denotes the weapon to use, for example, at extreme short range the shoulder, head butt and elbows work best. At medium range, the hammer fists and palm strikes work well and at longer range, the finger tip strikes and other movements done with moving in work very well.

Learning to conceal, draw and use weapons and improvised weapons is an essential bio-mechanical skill.

IX.   Launch positions

Work and become familiar with all the various launch positions:

Hands down
Hands up elusively whilst talking
Hands moving naturally
From various covert guards
From various covert moving guards
Also train your instinctive weapon drawing skills from various
concealments.

X.   Deceptions, voicing, distraction

Without these methods your techniques are simply techniques and
will lack 50% of what they could be.

In any combat using deception is an essential skill. Develop your
own unique repertoire of deceptions, these could range from
certain verbal phrases from which to launch mid-phrase. This could
also be certain deceptive movements which are your very own
from which you learn to launch. They could also be certain methods
of using your gaze to distract and confuse and combined with
words possibly, this could serve to distract momentarily in the lead
up to a brutal pre-emptive attack.

Five – Commitment

I.   For survival

Without the primal survival instinct i.e. The commitment, you will lack the animalistic energy and focus to prevail. How can you overcome any adversity without commitment? The first time you are hit or feel dazed, without commitment you will be minded to give up. Commit to survive, commit to help others survive, commit to do the right thing. Cultivation of this primal animalistic survival instinct is essential. A human being cannot fight but an animal can. Women are closer to this primal instinct, try taking or attacking their offspring... and see what happens.

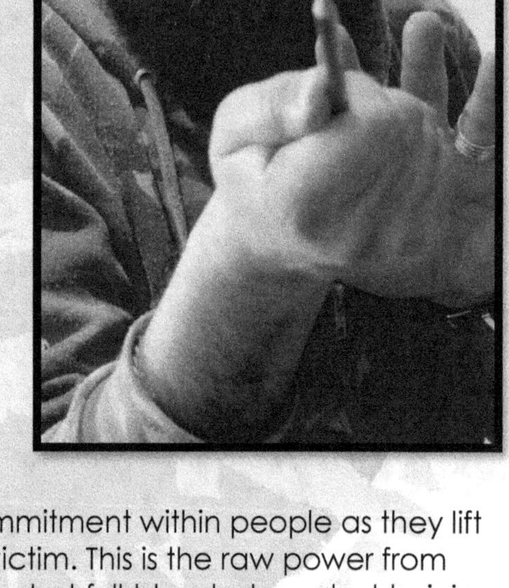

Similar examples are when loved ones are trapped under branches or vehicles, see the commitment within people as they lift extraordinary weight to free the victim. This is the raw power from total focused commitment. This is what full-blooded combat training seeks to bring out, refine and utilise.

II.   As a deterrence weapon to make them doubt themselves

When you see a dog and it suddenly turns crazy on you and starts snarling....and shows its' intent and commitment, how does that make you feel? Dogs sometimes do this for unexplained reasons but most animals do this as a protective warning mechanism. If an attacker senses, sees and hears true commitment in your eyes, posture, expression, movement, voice and energy, it will make him think again. Because it means that whoever wins, it's likely both parties will get injured. And this is not worth the risk. No one wants to fight a psycho. Psychos have no fear. They don't feel pain (until later) and they never stop. They can't be intimidated easily either. You need to portray you are a psycho. This is a temporary state. You're not really a psycho. But you need to learn to become one, firstly to deter your attacker/s and secondly to gain the extreme power that can only be harnessed in this state. The Chinese call this being more yang than the attacker.

III.   As a way to beat the debilitating affects of fear

Fear is often your own mind playing tricks on you by working against you. Learning to engage the primal instinct, immediately gives an outlet to the massive adrenaline dump accompanying the fight or flight mechanism. It is the human, logical, procrastinating mind which is your worst enemy in the moment of combat survival.

IV.   As a way to generate power

Over twenty years teaching experience has shown me that harnessing the attitude, commitment and emotional state can easily double the power of a strike. At a Qi or internal energy level, the power forges though the body and dynamically energises the system, it also makes the body far more resilient to pain from blows and more resistant to various types of damage which invariably results from a combat encounter.

Linking correct breathing to correct movement, posture, alignment, intent, commitment and energy transference certainly makes for a raw, explosive and powerful outcome.

V.   Solo training

The main objective of solo training is to train the mind to eliminate darkness and fear in day to day life and become aware of its debilitating and insidious affects upon you.

Eliminating this virus from your internal software will increase your potency in the Combat arena exponentially.

The other objectives of solo training are to deeply imbed reflective, natural, fluid and exclusive responses where you use the best weapon for the best target - which is normally a vital point, or a setup point combination leading to a vital point strike.

Train the mind to devise unpalatable and unpredictable scenarios that test you as a man ...or a woman.
Become familiar with these worst case scenarios. For example, imagine that you wake up to intruders and you are the only person standing between them and your sleeping loved ones.

Most of us live sanitised, safe, denatured lives, where we have been lead to strive for enslaved survival, by having to buy what was free and hankering for meaning and endless material comfort through carefully orchestrated educational and career paths. And we are taught to believe that others should and will protect us. This is all underpinned by media and advertising.

The unquestioned compliance to the system renders many incapable of feeling that deep animalistic commitment to effect the survival of oneself, one's family, one's clan.

An important element of your solo training is to realise the necessary control system within which you live and to take steps to stop the constant and insidious bombardment and brainwashing that seeks to control and emasculate by making you FEARFUL.

Also recognise that many sports masquerading as martial arts are nothing more than acrobatics, gymnastics or watered down martial derivatives designed to satisfy our need for combative pastimes, without ever changing us from the core and re-implanting and re-awakening our true instincts, intent and commitment.

Here's an easy hack. Turn off the television thus not allowing fear to be embedded in your heart. Lean to discern the real 'news'. Discern what is being misreported, under reported, not reported, over reported and what is being hidden, skewed or created for a wider agenda. There will be another book on solo training, the mind and escaping the shackles of implanted anxiety i.e. fear.

VI.   Progressive partner training

Learn to roll with and absorb slaps, punches and other contact, condition yourself to learn to deal with various undefended blows and strikes, accustom yourself to pain and desensitise yourself to any reluctance you may have towards being hit.
Armour up, get training buddies to attack you. Imagine in your mind a life threatening situation affecting your loved ones and then embed and utilise this committed mindset.

Progress to multiple attackers and weapons scenarios.

It is not the power you generate in partner work that is important, it is the mindset you learn and how you move and 'feel' inside. The power can be unleashed later.

VII. Pad and shield work

This is where you train full power and full contact, train as above, using single, multiple and multi-angular methods.

Ask your training buddies to motivate you by shouting at you with encouragement. Don't underestimate the power of collective training energy and team spirit.

Beast yourself with circuits immediately after a serious round of committed pad work.... Take yourself into unchartered uncomfortable territory. Don't beast yourself like this more than once a week.... If you do it right, you'll need time to recover and heal. The idea is to rip your lungs and body down and build them back stronger.

VIII. Pressure testing

This is where the attacker/s armour up, protect themselves as much as possible and really go for it. Work up to 'anything goes' from strikes to kicks, grabs and take downs and then weapons attacks too, move up to using improvised weapons, all be it mock up versions, to get the closest feel.

IX.   Self hypnosis / mental conditioning

Top athletes, gymnasts and boxers practice this. From positive thinking to full-on hypnosis and self hypnosis to internal suggestions implanted through entering a relaxed, receptive state where the mind and body can absorb and implement changes. Research this. It's real. Find a credible, vouched-for practitioner with at least twenty years experience, who teaches hypnosis, don't just find someone on the internet.

X.   As applied to internal dialogue and confidence

How far will you ever get if you don't believe you CAN, or WILL be, able to do something? Not very far.

We all have an internal dialogue or voice. We talk to ourselves all the time, in words and thought and beliefs. Change 'I can't' to 'I CAN'. 'I won't be able' to 'I WILL be able to', 'I can never be as good as him' to - 'he CAN so I CAN.'

Then forge your training and development plan in concrete, not sand.... And blast through it, marking out and gaining confidence from achieved goals and critical benchmarks in your progress. Gain power and confidence from your successes and your incremental progress, however small.

We learn and progress at different rates, at different times, progress can be up and down, a lumpy route. Not linear or as you'd think. Sometimes / often, we even have to invest in loss. We need to go back to go forward ! This is the difference between the world class practitioner and the mediocre wannabe.

The desire and commitment for progress is at a different level for some. These people welcome adversity in their training. And their egos, whilst often large, are suitably placated towards the greater objective of ultimate mastery.

Six - Stopping Power, breathing, voicing.

I.   Hit THROUGH - not at

This is a point of great importance for beginners and also advanced combatants.

Hitting at the target will not normally cause a stoppage or lasting debilitating damage. The exception to this is when advanced pressure point strikes or eye strikes are used, when glancing blows and medium force strikes can certainly do the job. The training needed to affect these methods is not to be underestimated and normally involves finding a reputable
master and practicing ancient arts to the point of near obsession.

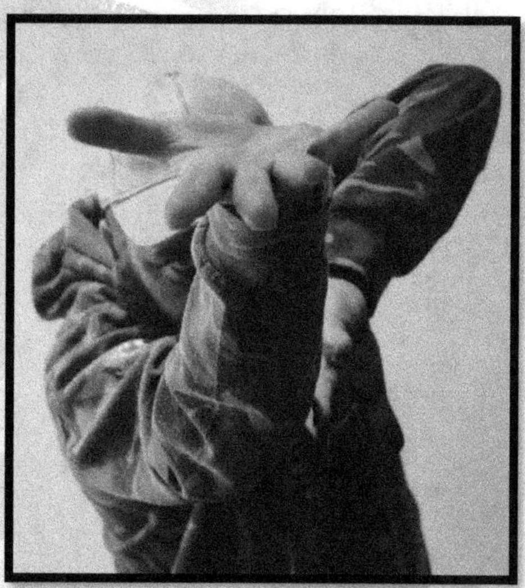

Or learn the MARA Combat system.

When one learns to strike through and not at, the effort needed to affect penetrative damage is far less and almost becomes like a committed touch or a committed movement as opposed to a blow per se.

II.   Use the whole body to generate power

This is the secret for normal sized or smaller people to be more powerful than much larger people or enemies. The sum of the whole will always be larger...

I have taught many smaller people and females and invariably they end up more powerful than their larger peers. Until the larger peers get a shock and then start listening and then in turn double or treble their own power. I once taught this to a student who was six feet four tall and eighteen stone. Initially, after a few months of training he caught up to me and we were both the same power and this stunned him somewhat as I am forty percent lighter and only five feet eight....and a half. After a couple of years of training his power was off the scale and only two people at my club could hope to hold the shields for him. This was the culmination of whole body movement, correct alignment, correct breathing and correct commitment and attitude. And much more in terms of internal energy power training, corrective diet and forms practice.

III.   Understand distancing and closing

Change your height, your head position, your distancing. Be elusive. Move in at angles and destroy. Adopt the elusive moving guard. Watch boxers.

Close the gap with your side, with your back to them, as well as to the front and at defined angles. Work this on the shields, pads and with partners.

Get your partner/s to be out of range, slightly, grossly and in between...and then practice pre-emptively moving into them. The objective being to intercept their attack and their intention.

Learn to watch the triangle between their forehead and shoulders, this should give you the best indication of their intention in terms of the method they might be planning to use, this is however always a risky business because people can easily change their minds and also use rapid combinations that render any of your defensive plans futile. It is for this reason that you must attack, the best defence offence !

Blocks don't work. And in MARA we steer clear of orthodox punches and kicks. Instead we favour various entry methods, guards and other body weapon attacking that could be mistaken for defence (with some wild clawing) to the uninitiated.

IV.   Inhale and explode

You need to breathe. So, if you can't live for more than a few minutes without oxygen and if your brain uses around eighty percent of your oxygen at any given time, then imagine what you can do if you can dramatically improve the uptake, quality and quantity of said oxygen.

In addition to lots of controlled breathing, Qi Gong energy work and daily woodland deep breathing and training, if you simply learn to inhale prior to any strike and then explode your breath out during any strike, you should double your power easily. I can normally quadruple a students power through stance, breathing and correct posture.

Breathe in with the nose to the lower belly area, aka the lower dantien in Chinese medicine or the hara in yogic understanding. Then explode with an aggressive 'HAA' sound as you strike, this should be the case for up to three or so strikes that launch explosively as a combination. This should be trained as part of your preemptive repertoire and methodology.

V.   Use the blood curdling warrior yell

This is like having an extra limb. So, you have the hands and feet.
Great. What about the fingers, thumbs, wrists, forearms, elbows,
shoulders, head, teeth, back, legs, knees, shins... And voice. In
ancient full blooded killing styles everything was identified, isolated
and honed as a weapon to fight and destroy. The voice is a serious
weapon, it fuels your intent and sends a primeval encoded
command to your central nervous system that this is for real ! It raises
the Qi. It's fires up the animal within you.
Similarly, it sends a disturbing message to your would-be attacker/s
that all is not as they had predicted. And that you have, in a
heartbeat, become a fearless, illogical, rabid animal who will fight
to the death. Dogs do this. So do wild animals. We have forgotten or
become too civilised.... Relearn this essential weapon.

VI.   Work on multiple attacks

Take your time in learning and perfecting drills where you have
multiple attacking partners and you perfect the timing and
distancing to affect a potentially deadly strike or telling blow. This
need not be actually driven through due to health and safety of
your partners. It's more about the potential and correctness of your
training.

VII. Solo drills

The best three things, for your overall power, that you can do solo
are: breathing, Qi gong energy work and forms practice, augment
this with club training.

For extreme power learn to move naturally... Be in a state of natural
balance and power all day, in everything you do. Practice honesty
and integrity, it would appear that practicing the 'warrior way'
invites positive power, whereas unethical practices and habits bring
only dis-ease and ultimately no joy, happiness or success.

VIII. Partner drills

Get your partners to armour up and practice pre arranged
sequences to strike the body armour full power, this will take some
training on the part of the partner to be able to withstand the strike -
even with armour on. For example, enter with an elbow spike to the
sternum, absorb with head guards of various types and then unleash
a portion of your power to their head (they are wearing a helmet!).

IX.   Pad and shield work

Round after round of tenacity fuelled pad and shield work is the
way forward. Never hit unless it's with full impact. Use all the breath,
body power, tenacity, animal instinct and remember to use the
proper follow through and distancing. Add the warrior cry and
you're working well.

X.   Combat circuit training and Pressure testing

Augment your power with all the afore mentioned methods,
combat circuit training can certainly assist too. In MARA we use
various Combat circuit methods, e.g. the dive bomber and others.
We use military push ups, core work, various planks and a multitude
of abdominal training. Judicious weight training, with light to
moderate weights, utilising whole body movements and never
isolating the muscle, will send a powerful message to the system.
Occasionally lift heavy. Work up to this and still only use full body
motions, cheat a bit don't damage yourself, especially your back.

Seven - Stopping points

Jaw

Struck with a lateral hammer fist, the back of the palm, the palm or an elbow, this is your classic knock out. People recover well from this in the movies, less so in real life. The blow can often be fatal if the person is knocked out and hit their head as they fall.

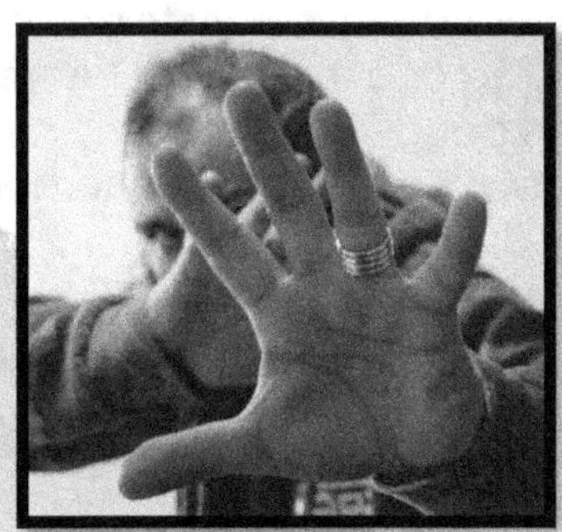

It is the shaking and displacement of the jaw that sends a signal to the brain that causes great local pain and knock out.

Neck

Hit anywhere on the neck and you'll get a result, even with medium force. With maximum force and with a powerful strike, for example an elbow, expect death to result. The neck is a vulnerable point because unlike the eyes / groin, there is no natural inbuilt flinch or defensive mechanism. The other classic strikes to the neck are with the knife hand strike, either upset, downward, or however made.

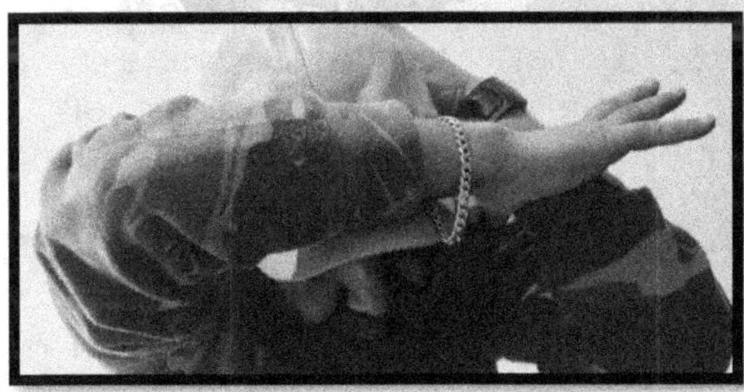

The various styles differ in how the knife hand is made and range from closed handed to open handed, slightly cupped to flat.

These are semantics and the Brit army was taught this strike back in ww2 as a method to kill the enemy. Many special forces have been taught this as a method of killing or a method of last resort. It works. It's dangerous, it doesn't need any set up points, the neck is vulnerable for the reasons outlined. The classic set up point would be on the inner wrist about three fingers up and is known as pericardium 6 in Chinese acupuncture.

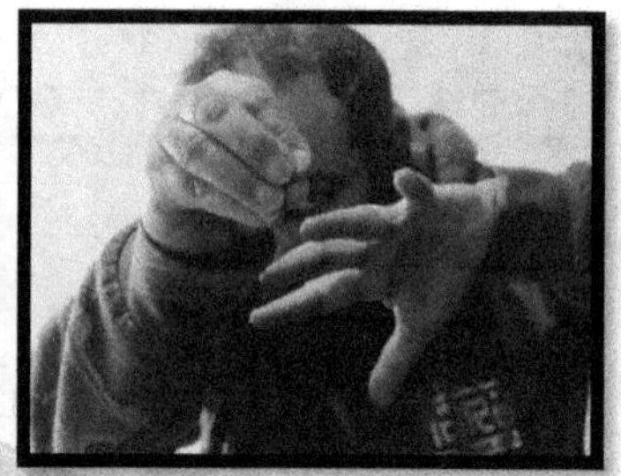

Back of head

Another potential kill shot. Even a light strike will cause dizziness and confusion. A medium strike will normally knock out. A hard blow will likely kill. Remember that even a knock out shot can be lethal when people fall and hit their head on a corner, a pavement or a table edge. Strike with Knife hands, hammer fists, any elbow or even a cupped hand hard smack, all will do the job. In Dim Mark these points are sometimes called gallbladder twenty. Hit straight into the occipital cavity or slightly upwards for maximum affect to strike the points and send an unrecoverable shock wave into the brain. Striking the back of the head is dangerous because many of the automatic systems of the body, like breathing, heart rate and blood pressure are run out of this area. Practice movements and footwork with your partner that enables you to quickly and deftly traverse or spin to the rear of the enemy, so that these strikes can be launched without much defence by the attacker. Some ancient Chinese styles capitalise on this particular method, finding a good school is hard and many masters no longer know, or no longer teach, the lethal combative components of their arts. The health benefitting and detailed movement aspects of these arts can overwhelm and distract many masters and exponents, this quest for ultimate knowledge is often detrimental to simply taking a few quality methods and drilling them to affect lethality in life or death combat situations.

Temple

This is near the thinnest part of the skull and a sharp blow here will cause a knock out or death. Any one-knuckle type strike, a sharp hammer fist or even a power slap, will all do the job. Elbowing this point will almost certainly kill.

Precision is needed but accidental blows are common in street fights, with thugs throwing bare knuckle hay makers and landing on the temple area, whereby people inadvertently get killed and people go to prison. So, be warned.

Solar plexus

This is the body blow supreme in terms of fight stoppage and potential lethality. An outward facing mid range palm strike is a covert explosive surprise shot, as is the verticle floating fist strike, which is essentially the same as the famous Bruce Lee one inch punch (which for real application normally travels around 6 inches) For a more lethal approach, the elbow spike or even the normal forearm elbow strike, will both do the job, especially when struck repeatedly in a machine gun like manner.

The solar plexus is known as the body brain in Traditional Chinese Medicine, as it is responsible for regulating many internal body processes, the physical damage from a strike is also tremendous as is the shock to the diaphragm and the resultant inability to draw in air. This damage and winding affect leaves the attacker nullified and open to further finishing blows to the temple or back of the head as they bend over or collapse.

Knee

Many energy meridians pass through the knee area, mainly on the sides and the back. On the inside we have the spleen and stomach meridians and on the back the kidney. These points cause extreme pain and internal damage, especially a sharp backward low stomp kick to the rear of the knee. Do not underestimate the long term internal kidney damage. Physically, the crushing affect of such a kick is obvious. A similar outcome can be achieved from a turbo charged take down, where you slip your foot covertly behind theirs and then suddenly straighten your knee to smash into the rear of theirs.

Other similarly dangerous and debilitating methods involve cutting your enemy down like a tree, by using your cross stomp kicks or angular knee strikes, this time into the sides of their knee. This snaps ligaments and collapses the joint, again causing pain, disablement, internal damage and rendering them open to lethal follow ups to the side of the neck, the temple and the back of the head.

Eyes

It doesn't really matter how big they are, a surprise strike to the eyes should do the job. It's hard to fight if you can't see and have searing pain in your eye socket. Pressure points under the eyes include a dangerous point called stomach one, clawing down under the eyes hits this point and causes extreme pain and internal damage that really is quite exquisite and unexpected. This is advanced dirty fighting par excellence.

To affect successful and affective eye strikes ones needs to develop explosive energy striking at light speed. The eyes have a God given natural reflexive flinch protection, hitting them is therefore a challenge. Finger strikes are the answer, launched with fluidity and where your strike reflexively finds its way via 'laser guided' stealth methodology.

Other surprise attacks to the eyes include the sideways finger tip slice, the downward raking claw and various one knuckle and thumb gauging methods.

Base of spine

Access the rear side of the attacker and affect a sharp upward knee to the lower spine. Increase the power and affect by dragging the head backward by the forehead or any other method. Make sure you don't get head-butted by them in the process, by mistake.

A classic method is to elbow the kidneys to cause internal bleeding and a slow debilitating demise.

Another method is to affect a full power double outward Palm strike to the kidneys. Similar affect as previously mentioned.

Obviously any stomp or kick to the lower spine when the enemy is already face down on the floor, will likely disable or likely kill. In WW2 British soldiers were taught to affect a double footed jumping donkey stomp onto the prostrate enemy to affect a kill.

Point of chin

This is an immediate knock out shot, which can kill if the attacker hits their head on the way down.

In MARA we use the downward hammer fist and downward backfist to great affect. The upward palm strike can also cause immediate stoppage as can any elbow strike.

High kicks are not recommended, due to the inherent dangers to your balance and other vulnerabilities caused; but can work too, if you're lucky.

Bridge of nose

This is a lovely shot as the nose explodes, the eyes water uncontrollably and the pain is immense. In MARA we use the downward palm heel strike and the downward hammer fist mainly. Other unique goring elbow digs can do the job and disfigure

permanently, if the enemy survives.
In MARA we have many unorthodox elbow methods, which are a
great surprise as they are little known outside the style.

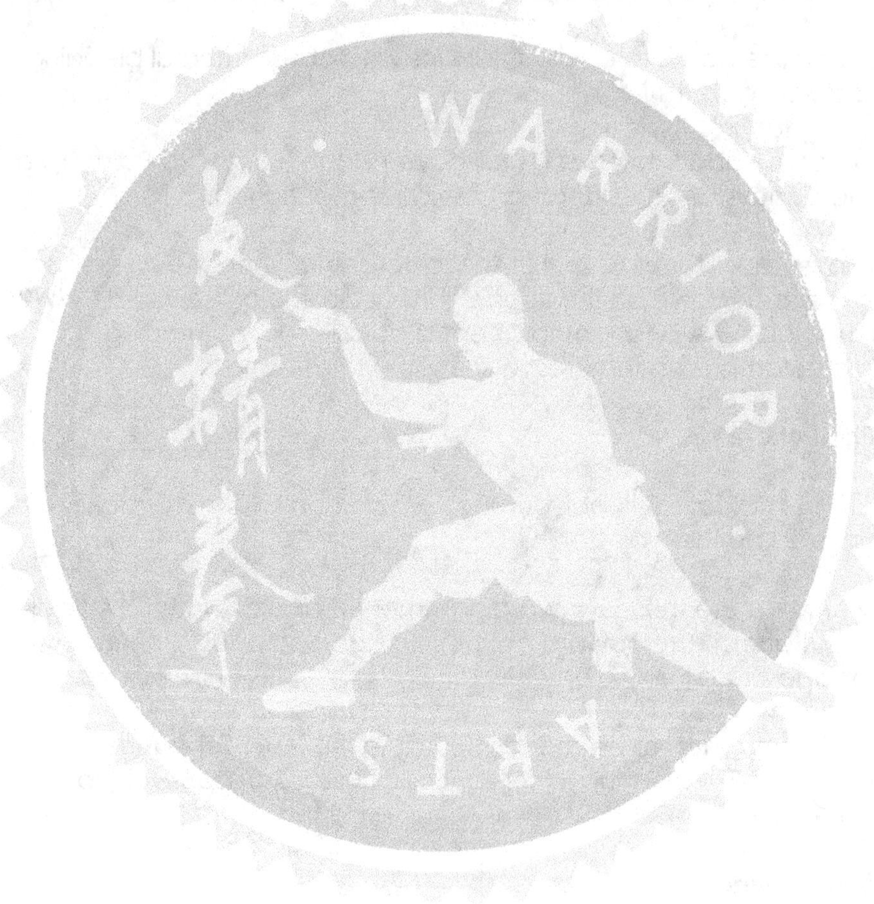

Eight - Improvised weapons

I.   The improvised weapon mindset

In MARA we train conventional combat weapons to gain the weapons mindset, this is useful for both empty handed and improvised weapons work.

Working with weapons also gives you the mindset to understand how weapons work and how you might in turn be attacked with weapons.

This area of training is not simple and learning from the uninitiated, inexperienced or misinformed will be significantly counter productive.

Weapons tend to operate most effectively in a smooth flow, which in turn leads to rapid fire usage and when this is applied in a covert and stealthy method, things get deadly. Knives and sticks are anything but crude implements and must be treated with the utmost respect.

Anything can be an improvised weapon, from an umbrella to a pen to a mobile phone to simple dirt, to an inane tea cup. Chairs and keys are weapons par excellence.

If you are attacked by someone with a knife and you have a chance to arm yourself with an improvised weapon, your chances of survival are likely to increase dramatically.

The extra reach from your weapon, coupled with the fact that you can possibly hit the knife-holding hand with less risk to you, will up your survival chances considerably. There is also the fact that you can affect deadly force with a sharp, blunt or hard object, improvised or otherwise.

The majority of knife attacks are covert and you won't know you have been sliced or stabbed until later, this is clearly a concern, you simply have to increase your awareness and enhance the way you live generally. Luck also plays a great part.

Improvised weapons are only any good if you have the chance to use them. And if they are at hand. And you have the skill and reflexive responsiveness ingrained to get to them, use them and not drop them under pressure. And fear doesn't get the better of you and allows at least your gross motor functions to operate with what has been ingrained under pressure.

Ok, so, you're interested in improvised weapons, you live in a very civilised country where all the criminals carry weapons and all the law abiding tax paying schmuks don't carry because the law has banned them from doing so. How very civilised.

The UK, parts of Europe and other lovely places have all banned even most rudimentary of <u>self defence tools</u>. So, what are you left with? Not much? Nope. The world is your lobster as they say…. You are limited only by your own imagination. I actually think that because of their stealth, improvised weapons are potentially more shocking than conventional weapons, thankfully not many know this.

II.   How to train for improvised weapons

Learn combat knife, combat stick and combat cane.

Then, once you have learned the basics to a competent level, create your own repertoire of what works for you. Then apply this to your favourite improvised weapons, that work for you, your hand shape and size.

Learn to bond with your chosen weapon/s. Hold them, caress them, feel them. Yes, I know this sounds a bit odd but it's what you need to do.

III.   Solo

Learn to draw the weapon.

Decide where you will keep each weapon type, e.g. Keys will always be in your right pocket, phone will always be in your left pocket, the oversized bottle opener will always be in your inside pocket etc.

Then learn to make the draw meld into the attack, so you have a seamless draw and attack.

Learn to draw with stealth. So that your movements appear natural and are cloaked, not telegraphed.

Learn to obscure the enemies eyes with slaps, covers and other measures, just before attack, these are designed to increase your chances of successful delivery of the tool you are using, be whatever that may be.

IV.   Partner drills

Do all of the above but with a partner and then partners to replicate multiple opponents. Do this with empty handed attacks and then with them having weapons too.

Explore all the scenarios you can think of and utilise different environments and different lighting. Then do the same but add pre-exhaustion into the mix to increase the pressure and to replicate the debilitating effects of fear.

Start the multiple opponent work with their attacking weapons stationary or held in a threatening manner.

Work up to their weapons moving slowly, then moving faster and at different angles of attack.

Keep things safe by using safe replica weapons for the attack and defence, if you can't buy any, then make some using light wood covered with soft foam pipe insulation. I have made perfectly workable training weapons with cardboard and insulating tape !

V.   Power training and flow training

Learn about power striking with improvised weapons like umbrellas and various sticks by working up to full power on the tyres. Buy an unbreakable training stick, like Chinese bamboo or super hard ratan, some polypropylene training sticks are also very tough. Then whack the hell out of a hanging tyre. Don't over reach and make

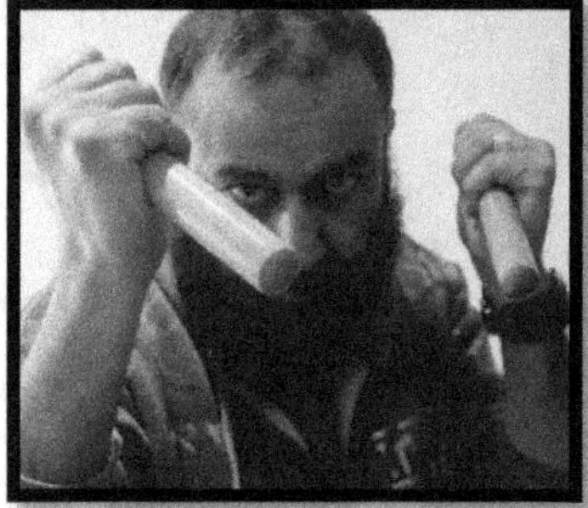

sure you control the weapon on your centre line. Dont flail. Be controlled. Use your wrist and other joints to transfer power.

For flow, learn about small circle knife work from advanced martial arts or study a credible military combat knife style.

MARA has its own combat knife drills and forms to teach this. Once learned this can be easily applied to any small sharp improvised weapons such as pens, letter openers, bottle openers, certain mobile phones, scissors and anything else you can think of.

VI.   Keys and other sharp objects

Keys - these can be used for stabbing, slashing, gauging or punching, they can be held in a variety of ways ranging from e.g. held between the thumb and forefinger, or flailing from a long chain or hand held keyfob. Check our <u>Instagram</u> page for demos of certain key fob holders (<u>tactikey</u>) that are great for enhancing the effect.

Attacking the eyes with keys is always a good strategy as are other
dirty methods whereby short stabs / jabs are inflicted into the
floating ribs and other low line vulnerable areas.

VII. Umbrellas and other stick like objects

Attacking the knees and outer thigh with powerful inward or
outward blows is a great strategy, flowing into seamless downward
follow ups to their head as they are on the way down is clearly a
lethal strategy and reserved for life or death scenarios.

Don't neglect the power of the two handed method, with has the
advantage of a safer grip and being able to affect powerful
upward strikes to the neck. The debilitating power of the double
handed butt strike is hard to describe when affected against the
solar plexus or any other part of the enemy's body. Using double
handed strikes in a curve against the side of the head is another
lethal fight stopper and is again reserved for life or death scenarios.

VIII. Phones and other blunt objects

Virtually any object in the right hands is a
potentially dangerous implement or improvised
weapon. This is the case with any small handheld
hard object, mobile phones, cups, mugs,
ornaments, candle holders and any other small
wooden or hard plastic object.

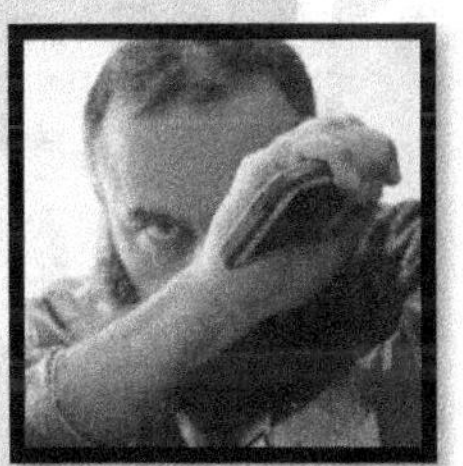

IX. Pens / pencils / chopsticks / torches / screwdrivers / scissors.

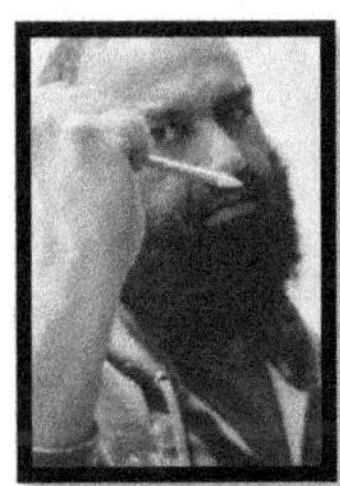

If security is tight and checks are in place (but you still
fear high risk), then go no further than your common or
garden, humble and simple sharpened wooden pencil.
Or pen. Or plastic highlighter. Or even a chopstick or
two. As stabbing weapons they are unparalleled for
their sheer simplicity and every day availability and
acceptability.

Learn to hold these objects between the forefinger and thumb, securely wedged in, so that the thumb muscle in your hand creates a nice support.

Straight line, low level stabs work well, against the ribs, kidneys, liver or in through the ribs like an ice pick into the heart, neck or other vitals.

Don't underestimate the ramifications of a neck stab in terms of attention from the police and on lookers. Save this one for life or death, military applications or when shock and awe is desirable, e.g. When multiple opponents or weapons are being utilised against you, or when criminals are in your home, threaten lethality or molestation against your loved ones and you want to give them something to think about.

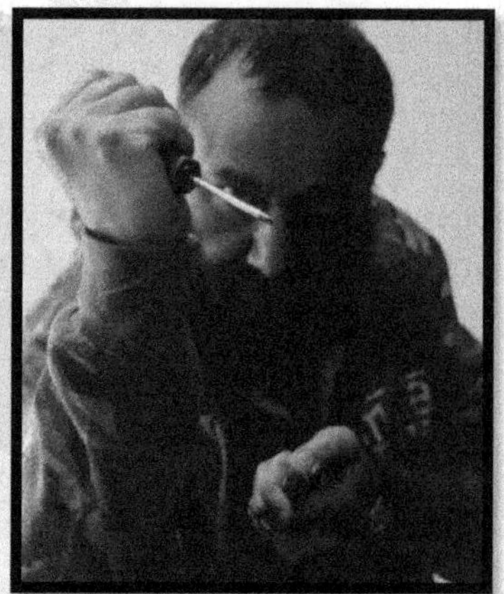

Adding a slight curve to your movements with the pen can also be a big shock, assuming they haven't even noticed your covert improvised <u>weaponary</u>, the reverse waist turn is also a lovely shocker, this is when you turn in the opposite direction to the strike as you shoot out the pen (or similar) into their eye, throat etc. Check my <u>Instagram</u> for trials on various carbon fibre non metallic 'tools'.

X.   Covert tactics, deception and speed

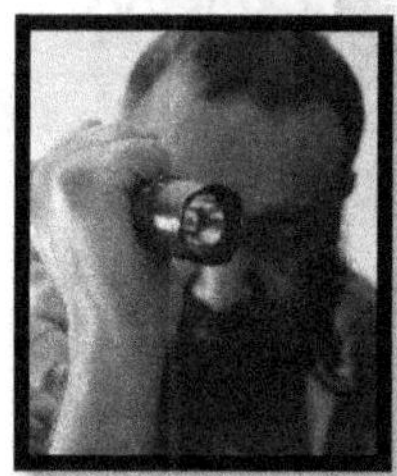

As mentioned, keep your improvised weapons in specific pockets and places. Learn to draw them and use them. Cover their eyes if possible prior to the main attack and practice increasing speed, until you become explosive, fluid and irresistible. I.e. Almost impossible to defend against.

Learn to get close, by stealth and to draw and stab at almost point blank range, so it's too late… and they don't know what's happened until they feel the dull pain and see the warm blood on their clothes or hand. Before they collapse, from either shock, blood loss or internal bleeding.

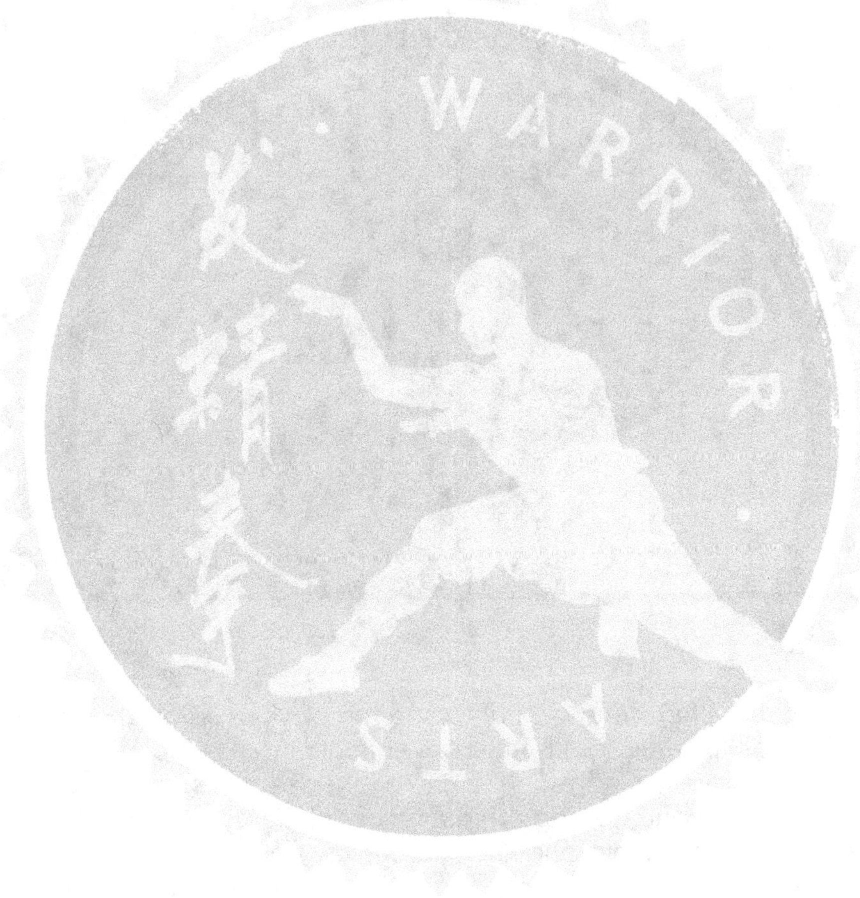

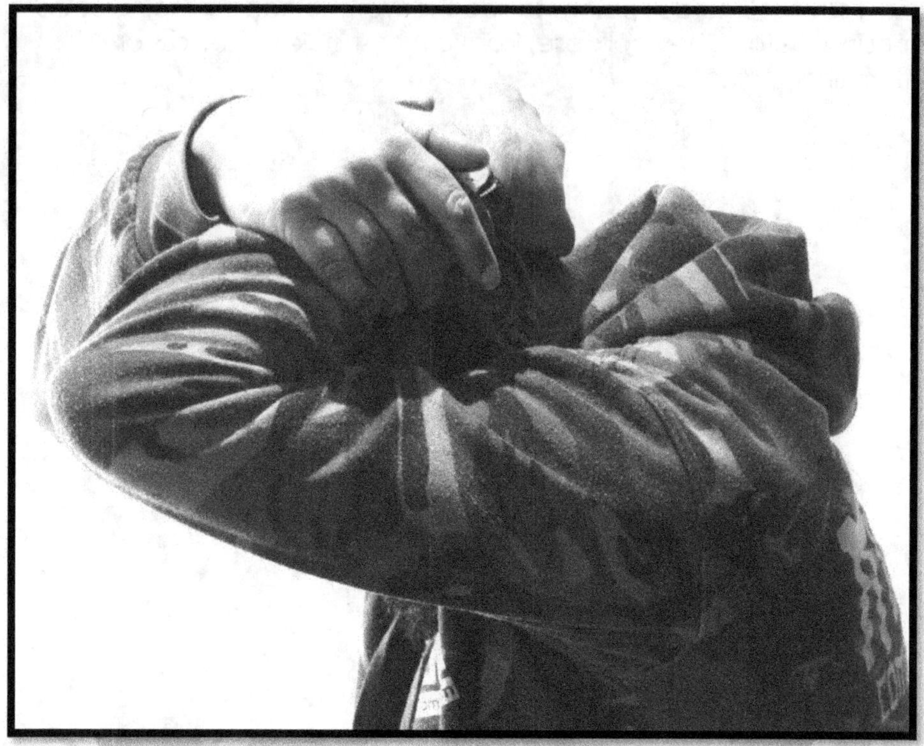

I.   **Fist**

This is a matter of preference but for me the obvious (wrong) choice (in a life or death situation) is the conventional fist. The main fists used in MARA are the hammerfists, in various directions, downward, inward, outward and flowing off the various head guards. We do however also use various one knuckle punches, like the tiger paw and the Phoenix fist and also the jaguar fist, these are made using the middle knuckle, forefinger knuckle and full set of secondary knuckles. These are lethal and targeted at the eyes, neck, throat and temple and some vulnerable abdominal areas too.

In MARA, we are fans of the Bruce Lee one in punch (which, when applied is actually a six inch power blast), or vertical floating explosive fist. It is speedy, powerful and is an advanced martial movement. Obvious targets for this are the solar plexus. But in MARA we tend to target the area between the eyes, the cheek bone, the eye socket, behind the ear and the dangerous liver accu points under the pec / chest muscle.

Other punches include the infamous MARA hollow fist.

From the classics we have the secret dog fist method, which utilises a last second turning action of the fist when strike the temple with the last three knuckles.

II. Fingers

Any classical or neo classical full blooded killing style will be utilising the fingers to strike (and claw and gauge) the eyes and throat, these methods necessitate some conditioning and know how about how to make the various spear hand strikes and the fingers generally, once learned, conditioned and embedded, these methods give you a loaded gun at your finger tips.

Some styles make the spear hand with closed straight fingers, others with closed slightly curved fingers, in Ninjitsu it's slightly different with only three fingers being used and the thumb and little finger touching.

In some ancient classics from China they tend to use the index and middle fingers in a cobra strike. In MARA we use the open handed, open fingers, in a strong resilient rake, or straight into the eyes. In some circles this is also known as the Dim Mak claw.
Bruce Lee was a great advocate of the lead finger jab and the knee stomp as he preferred these as openers.

Work these strikes on a light focus mitt, held lightly, or on hung news paper. Which you can increase in thickness as you become more adept.

Used both preemptively and as an attack after entering, the fingers to the eyes are a fight stopper par excellence. Used with even slightly conditioned fingers to the throat or sides of the neck they are dangerous indeed.

In discussing finger strikes we will include the thumb gauge to the eyes as having equal potency to cause an abrupt and painful stoppage and cessation in motivation for the would be attacker.

III.   Elbows

If you have no time or are a beginner then you would do best to work your elbows. In all directions and on the heavy bag. And in a multitude of methods. They can be used offensively, to enter, to withstand attacks by protecting your own vital areas and to cause dramatic stoppage.

An entire DVD has been devised solely on how elbows (and forearms) are used in MARA. We like elbow strikes so much we have named them with exotic names ! Like the Butterfly elbow, the Rhino, the Pick Axe. We love them all.

Here are some key pointers:

Try and protect your head and neck as much as possible by launching elbows in such a way that they wrap around your head, with your chin tucked in. Avoid peering over. Be crouched, cloaked and compact.

Contemplate the various elbow methods and the various entry methods, which in turn should roll onto various natural strikes and finishes.

This is what MARA is all about. Covert dramatic, preemptive entry, rapid fire strikes launched elusively from the entry guard and continuance of fully committed explosive striking until the threat is subdued or we have escaped.

Don't cock the elbow back, this telegraphs your intention. Instead, learn how to generate power from correct structure and by using the full body to generate power.

IV.   Forearms.

These are often known as elbow strikes, but the true forearm strike is a vicious rotating beast of the highest order and is used as a short range blast into the neck. Adding rotation and an upward motion serves to inflict the most internal damage as does adding an inward angle into the neck and out of the other side. This type of strike is a direct application (as are many other strikes) of your Qi Gong postures.

V.   Knees

These are the best short range power tools to affect bone crunching stoppage. Everything is a target for these hugely boney and well muscled fearless friends.

Once you have entered and given him something to think about, using any of the afore mentioned methods, finishing with a swift graceful knee to his head, body, inner or out thighs or the side of his knee, adding a jumping element will cause great shock, surprise and will turbo the power by about double.

In MARA the knees are used as a straight in dig, with a joining elbow to bounce into the target, upward or inward and even outward.

VI. Head

Being a heavy and well boned structure, the head clearly has potential as a weapon, not generally used in sport martial arts because of its unpredictable and brutal impact. The head has to be understood in order to cause maximum damage to the enemy - not to you, there is little worse than knocking yourself out !

Use the well structured top of the forehead or the bony hard back of the head. Don't use the temple or any thinly boned or sensitive areas, test this for yourself lightly to learn about your head structure.

Blasting upward, sideways or downward, into the enemies face or temple is a great strategy at close range, as is using the back of the head in bear hug or rear attack scenarios. Head butting the sternum or solar plexus also createS space at close range and can wind the enemy, opening them up for more dramatic finishes with pouding hammer fists and downward elbows.

VII. Shoulder

A lot of martial arts neglect this strike, most real combat arts and contact sports know about the efficacy of the shoulder strike. It can be used to take the enemy off his feet and to cause stoppage by affecting a downward penetrative shoulder blow to his sternum / breast plate area.

Always combine shoulder strike training with a proper understanding of how you need to protect your own neck and head at close range. Keep your chin down and use your rear hand to simultaneously protect your face. This is a point blank method for ultra close range usage only. Following up with a head butt and then wrapping their head onto a finishing knee works wonders

VIII. Teeth

Weapons of last resort as no one wants to catch something nasty, biting is reserved for when it's all gone terribly wrong, bite their ear off, bite their cheek, or anything you can. This is for extreme grappling situations e.g. where his compadres want to stamp on your head and you need to escape fast.

Biting can also be used in extreme stand up grappling, when you have been clinched and are being bear hugged to the point of having no breath left or when you have him in a head lock and want to cause an emotional disturbance to the other attackers, to show them you are crazy and that fighting with you is an undesirable and dangerous endeavour. Do get a blood test afterwards.

IX. Feet

Knowing how to use the feet is essential, you will normally be wearing shoes of some type, so for combat training definitely wear shoes or trainers. The fight stopping methods to his legs / inner thighs / outer thighs / knees will include the heel stomp, the toe jab and the shin swing. Your boots are a weapon. Don't understimate the advantage gained from power kicks and downward scrapesand stomps, inflicted to his foot or shin whilst wearing heavy shoes or boots.

In MARA we use normal kicks sparingly, this is due to our own balance and rooting being prioritised and that in multiple opponent and weapons scenarios a judicious and cautious approach is desirable.

X. Grabbing and tearing.

It takes only around nine pounds of downward ripping force to tear an ear off.

Showing your power in grabbing and tearing can traumatise a would be attacker and their gang, the pain and disfigurement will certainly be a deterrence.

Ten - Blocks, kicks, punches, head guards and entry methods.

I. Forget about blocks, kicks and punches

Not withstanding that we mentioned kicks and punches above, these will not be your bread and butter methods, AT ALL, unless you know how to use them appropriately, judiciously and in the special manner outlined.

Forget about the movies.

And forget the vast majority of 'expert' demos you might see against compliant training partners demonstrated at long range.

Here are some better ideas:

II. Head guard entry methods, why, how, insurance policy.

Basically, these are methods to cover your head and enter quickly and powerfully and is the ultimate body weapon sting operation.

Focus on developing ease in the use of these methods as they will give you an advantage which is unfair.

These methods are somewhat like putting the game in 'cheat mode'. Simply enter with these, then immediately launch your attack and enjoy the fun. An attack after entry which utilises your hands in a never ending rotating, tearing clawing method to the eyes and face can stun and startle. And affect suitable openings to finish the enemy.

Key errors include standing still with the head guard on, the enemy will work out your strategy in a heart beat and change tack to exploit your exposed weaknesses.

Instead insure that your body is crouched, your head is down, have your chin in, move in directly or at an angle, use these methods as an ATTACK and you'll up your chances. Use them as defence and expect almost certain defeat.

III.   Moving in not stationary

Did I mention you need to move in ! Practice this at all angles and with various turns.

IV.   It's a weapon (the various entry methods).

Did I mention that an offensive mindset will work and a defensive one might not?

V.   Entry methods utilising the head guard and other methods

Entry methods are movements that allow you to move into ultra-close range of your opponent, invading his space, putting off his timing, thereby giving you an opening to unleash ferocious strikes.

But in MARA, their beauty is that they build on instinctive, reflexive movements that one might instinctively make when an attack is launched, such as raising your arms and lowering your head when a punch is thrown.

This reflex action has been embedded into an effective defence – "the Head Guard" – that becomes an aggressive counterattack when stepping into the opponent. Entry methods are one of the golden nuggets of MARA. These are not blocks, that would take years of dedicated practice (and even then would probably still not be fast enough). Blocks don't work very well in a real street fight, where rapid fire compound committed blows come at you from all angles.

In MARA we have several different types of head guards which are utilised as entry methods and weapons in their own right, they are offensive, to the uninitiated they may appear defensive. Often, the single most challenging aspect of the training for new initiates is our use of entry methods and head guards.

This area of training is specialist and requires proper instruction. The first aspect of the training is to learn how to put the various head guards on. The next part of the training is to use these with a move in action. The third part of the training is to work the guards against various attacks and strikes.

The final aspect of the training is to understand which strikes and other potent clawing methods can be reliably used immediately and naturally from the guard position. The MARA forms embed this aspect in particular.

Here is an introduction to the subject of head guards and entry methods in MARA.

Head guard one - double head guard - both hands up on the head, one over the other, close the forearms together head down, crouched position, use as a battering ram. Can be used against strikes or pre-emptively.

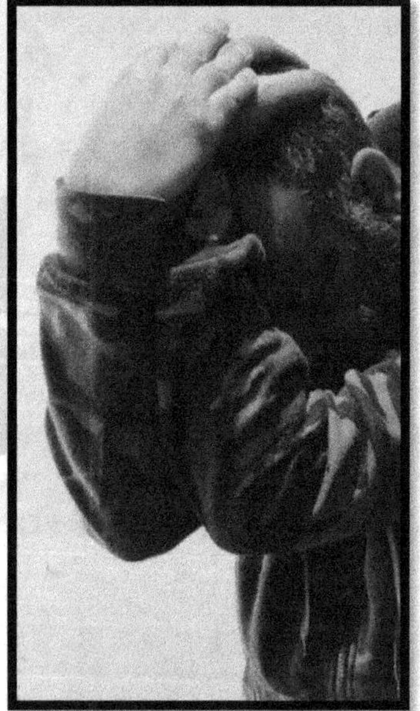

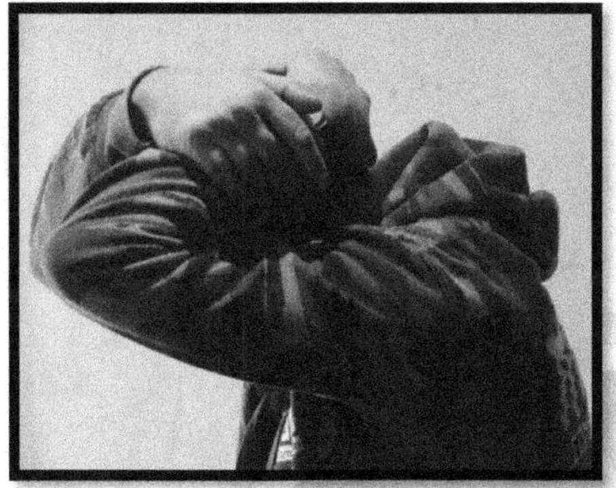

Head guard two - Single front head guard - can be done either on the right or the left, create this guard by putting the cupped hand behind the head and closing the forearm and elbow against the head with the other hand over the top.

Again, use against their strikes or pre-emptively against the head or body.

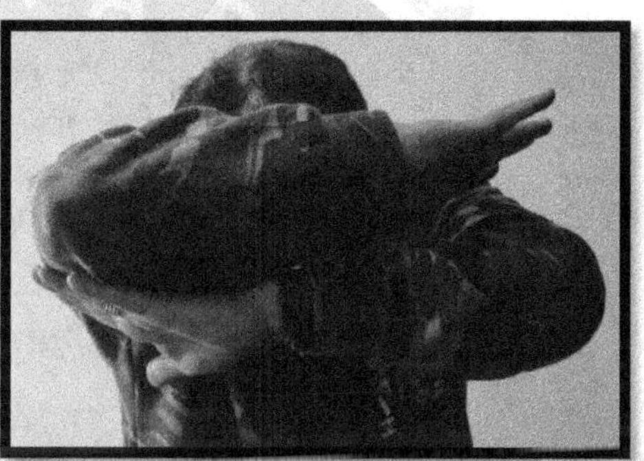

Head guard three - Single side/rear head guard - as above but used with a turn against side or rear attacks.

Head guard four - lateral head guard - this guard is created using both arms parallel in front of the face, from a crouched position and the chin tucked in peering through the middle. Again, use against their strikes or pre-emptively.

Head guard / knee - Single front head guard combined with jumping knee - this utilises a single head guard with the same side touching the elbow, the idea is to shift your body weight in towards the click for oncoming attack.

Please check our online shop for other detailed training manuals; our social media pages and <u>YouTube</u> channel also have regularly posted content demonstrating these methods.

VI. Solo training

This is done as forms, shadow work, on the bag and in free form.

The MARA forms have these various Head guards and entry methods embedded, subscribe to our channels on social media / <u>YouTube</u> and get hold of some MARA training material.

VII. Partner training

The above entry methods and head guards should be worked with a partner, initially with light contact, always using <u>gloves</u>, head guards and body armour available. Increase the intensity of the training in terms of contact, Single and multiple attacks, angles and directions and also multiple opponents. Finally, weapons can be also introduced into the training.

VIII. Pad and shield work

The various head guards and entry methods can be worked on focus mitts, Thai pads and large shields.

Again, check out <u>our books</u>, DVD's, social media and <u>YouTube</u> channel for examples of this type of training. In essence, you are limited by your own imagination.

IX. Common errors

Not moving in when applying these methods will leave you vulnerable, the enemy will soon work out your strategy and will pick you apart.

Not protecting the back of the head with the cupped hand. This is a particular error on the single head guard when students do not cover the back of the head, this leaves you vulnerable to swings and other attacks which may inadvertently or purposely targeted to the rear of your head.

Inadvertently leaving a gap that exposes your face is another dangerous strategy. This is particularly pertinent to the first head guard, this being a double head guard. For some reason students often get in the habit of leaving a large gap between the two forearms that exposes the face. As I always say - if you don't hear you will FEEL.

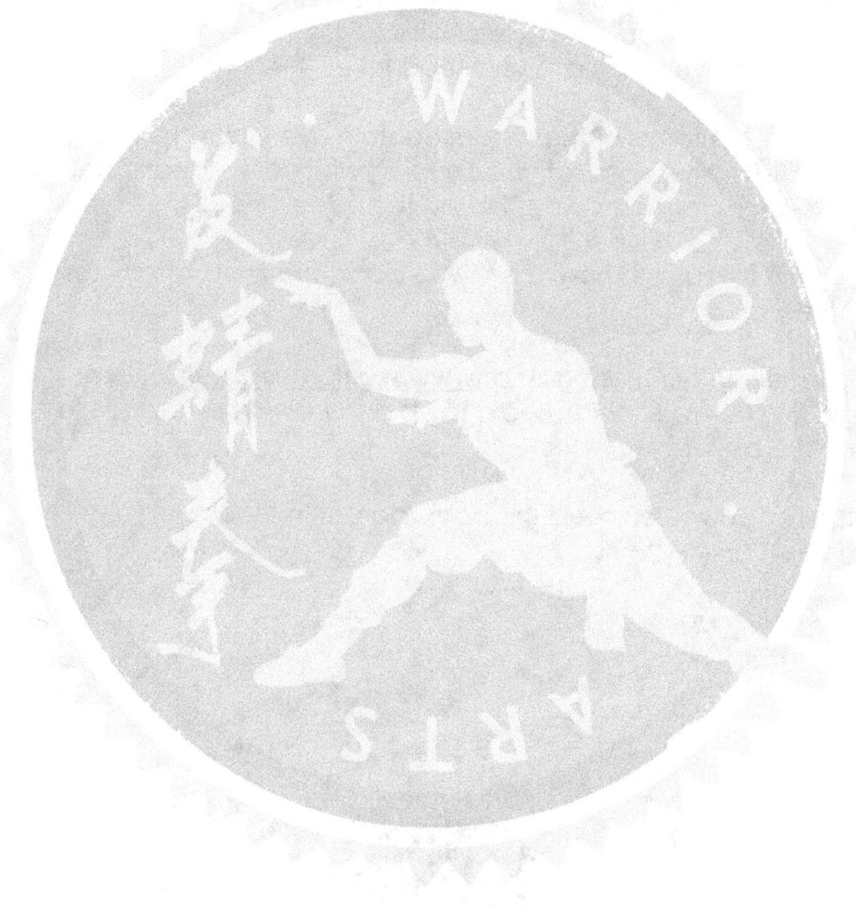

What comes next?
...The MARA forms and structured training programme

Well done and thanks, firstly for reading this book and hopefully secondly for trying out the methods. If you like what you have read and would like to take this further, then please take steps to learn the particular forms within the MARA system, these have been designed to give you the edge and to embed reflexive and dangerous movements into your repertoire.

The three core forms of the system contain everything you need to know for effective combat, this coupled with our weapons training and weapons forms should give you the edge.

The MARA forms are known as the 10 pack, The Mass Attack Drill and the LSM.

Put yourself on our mailing list at www.warriorarts.co.uk for our books, DVD's, Free Social Media posts and training packages to teach the above.

Finally, I hope you enjoyed this book, do get in touch with any comments or questions.

Peace and Love.

Dave V.

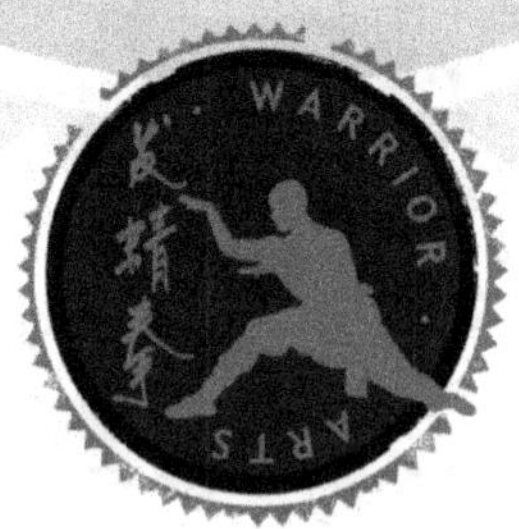

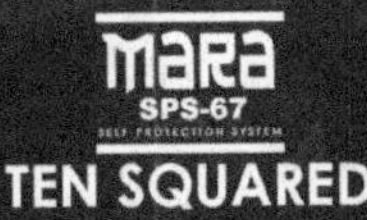

TEN SQUARED

The book is written in a relaxed, accessible and colloquial style. Those who have met Dave V, either personally or through his social media presence, can hear him speak in his inimitable style, whilst those who do not, quickly get to know him.

The book brings a wealth of wisdom that is beneficial to the general public as well as martial arts practitioners.

This work is especially valuable for those who truly want to be effective in real-life encounters and might otherwise undertake 'martial arts' under the false belief that it will serve them on the street or other no rules attack.

Ten Squared is for everyone who wants to take their safety seriously, and gain some genuine and effective solutions to real street violence. It's equally for Martial arts enthusiasts who need to understand real violence, and effective techniques to counter it.

Ten Squared aims to address the following objectives:

To bring about a mind-set change about personal safety: becoming streetwise, perceptive, prepared and sensible.

To make you understand the true mentality of thugs: the idea that there is no 'fair fight'

To give you a mindset, techniques and tools to be effective in real street fighting situations.

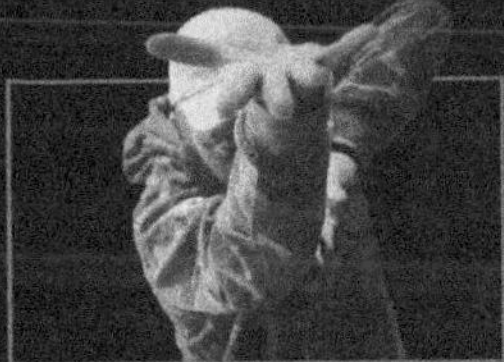

For more information and access to other ePublications from Dave V, please visit Warrior Arts online at

www.warriorarts.co.uk

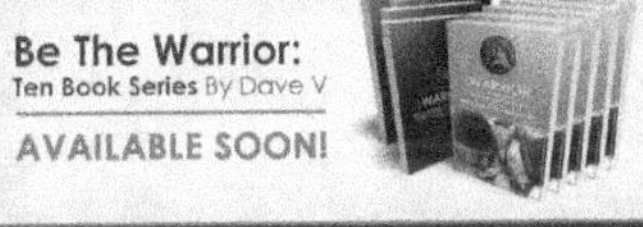

Written and published by founder and chief instructor, Dave V, the "Be The Warrior" series of books Builds on ideas in the TEN SQUARED book and also covers important aspects of the MARA syllabus.

Please visit the Warrior Arts website/online shop to learn more and purchase.

First Published: 2018
Revision 2 - 04/2018

www.ingramcontent.com/pod-product-compliance
Lightning Source LLC
Chambersburg PA
CBHW070033260726
48658CB00002B/617